The Longevity Bible

Also by Gary Small, M.D.

The Memory Bible

with Gigi Vorgan
The Memory Prescription

The Longevity Bible

8 Essential Strategies for
Keeping Your Mind Sharp and
Your Body Young

Gary Small, M.D.

with Gigi Vorgan

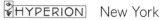 HYPERION New York

Photographs by Sterling Franken-Steffen. Model: Gigi Vorgan.

Library of Congress Cataloging-in-Publication Data

Small, Gary W.
    The longevity bible : 8 essential strategies for keeping your mind sharp and your body young / by Gary Small with Gigi Vorgan. — 1st ed.
        p. cm.
Includes bibliographical references and index.
ISBN 1-4013-0184-3
    1. Longevity. 2. Aging. 3. Health. I. Vorgan, Gigi. II. Title.

RA776.75.S565 2006
613.2—dc22   2005055114

Hyperion books are available for special promotions and premiums. For details contact Michael Rentas, Assistant Director, Inventory Operations, Hyperion, 77 West 66th Street, 12th floor, New York, New York 10023, or call 212-456-0133.

FIRST EDITION

10 9 8 7 6 5 4 3 2 1

We dedicate this book to our loving family,
especially our children,
Rachel and Harry.
Their sweet faces and enthusiasm
enrich our lives every day,
and make us grateful
for the quality of our longevity.

Contents

Contents

Contents

Acknowledgments

Many friends and colleagues provided valuable input and encouragement during the writing of this book, including Helen Berman, Susan Bowerman, Rachel Champeau, Susan Coddon, Neal Frankle, Dr. Martin Greenberger, Dr. David Heber, Dr. Robert Hucherson, Dr. Shirley Impellizzeri, Andrea Kaplan, Dr. Daniel Keatinge, Chef David Lawrence, Kimberly McClain, Dr. Michael Persky, Dr. Judith Reichman, Dr. Peter Rosen, Michele and Dr. Nathan Rubin, Dottie Sefton, Sandi Shapiro, Pauline Spaulding, and Cara and Rob Steinberg. We are also indebted to our talented photographer and friend, Sterling Franken-Steffen, and our publicists Grace McQuade and Lynn Goldberg, as well as our outstanding publishing team at Hyperion, including our wonderful editor Brenda Copeland; Zareen Jaffery; our tireless publicist Beth Dickey; and the rest of the Hyperion family. This book would not have been possible without the support of Mary Ellen O'Neill and our longtime agent and good friend, Sandra Dijkstra, whose talent and instincts never cease to amaze us.

Gary Small, M.D.
Gigi Vorgan

The Longevity Bible

Part 1

Quality Longevity—
Living Longer, Younger,
and Healthier

It is not enough to add years to one's life . . .
one must also add life to those years.

—JOHN F. KENNEDY

You're savoring your ritual cappuccino across the street from your dentist's office when this incredibly handsome young guy sits down two tables over. Your eyes meet his and he smiles seductively—you practically choke. You could swear you know him from somewhere. . . . He gives you a little wave. Where the heck could you know him from? He's so *young*. And you've been married a *long* time. Oh my god, he's coming over! Could this amazing hunk *possibly* be hitting on you? Ridiculous. No way! Thank God in heaven you just had your teeth cleaned. He grins broadly. "Hi! Remember me?!" You're completely at a loss. "I'm Andy! Andy Carter! I was on your son's basketball team in middle school." You freeze with a ridiculous smile on your face and a sudden urge to evaporate into thin air.

Age reminders happen to everyone. It could be as simple as the appearance of a single gray hair, the first time someone calls you "Ma'am," or perhaps walking into a room and forgetting the reason why. None of us can stop time, but we *can* slow down the effects of aging—and sometimes even reverse them.

A mere one hundred years ago, people were lucky to live beyond age forty. Now, life expectancy has risen to age seventy-four for men and eighty for women, and recent studies show that the average sixty-five-year-old American can expect to live another seventeen years. Modern medical science is striving to keep us alive well into our nineties and beyond, and most people say they want to live as long as possible. But who wants to live to be one hundred without their health, vitality, and faculties intact? That's where *The Longevity Bible's Eight Essentials* come in—showing us how to keep it *all* together—our brains, our bodies, and our attitudes.

The Eight Essentials

Traditionally, magazine and television advertisers have focused their marketing strategies on youthful looks and attitudes to attract consumers to their products. Recently, however, there has been a shift in tactics. Today, Madison Avenue's emphasis is not so much on youthful demographics but on "psychographics"—marketing focused toward the age group in which consumers actually *perceive* themselves as being. Try asking baby boomers how old they consider themselves, not in actual calendar years, but mentally and physically. Many will confess they still have the attitude of a twenty-five-year-old and feel nowhere near their chronological age.

Most of us protest against the idea of aging in the way our parents did and vow to fight against the process as long as possible. We are looking for a safe, convenient, medically sound way to live longer, empower ourselves, and remain healthy and fulfilled throughout that long life—what I refer to as "quality longevity."

Empowering ourselves for the future requires learning new skills, as well as honing the ones we already have. In my last book, *The Memory Prescription*, I showed how we could jump-start our brain and body fitness by focusing on four of the basic essentials:

achieving *mental sharpness, physical fitness, a healthy diet,* and *stress reduction.* Now, in *The Longevity Bible,* I outline my entire program—all Eight Essentials—to allow every one of us to achieve our own maximum, quality longevity in every area of our lives. These essential strategies include keys to *keeping a positive outlook, cultivating healthy relationships, getting the most out of modern medicine,* and *adapting and flourishing in a changing environment.*

We'll look at the science behind the Eight Essentials, and at simple and practical ways for integrating them into our daily life. When practiced together, these Eight Essentials create a synergy that achieves positive results faster and far more effectively than could be achieved by doing them individually.

Fix Your Brain First: The Rest Will Follow

We begin our longevity solution by sharpening our minds (Essential 1) and maximizing our brain fitness. Fix your brain for longevity, and your body will follow in kind. By keeping our minds sharp, we are more inclined to stay physically fit, enhance our relationships, maintain a longevity diet, and follow the other healthy lifestyle strategies outlined in this book. In fact, all the Essentials contribute to keeping our brains young, fit, and cognitively strong throughout all stages of life. Simply doing mental aerobics can significantly improve memory skills and, when combined with the other Essentials, may extend life expectancy. A recent study found that mentally stimulating leisure activities such as reading, doing crossword puzzles, or playing board games lowers the risk for Alzheimer's disease by nearly a third.

Scientific evidence shows that keeping a positive outlook (Essential 2) helps us to stay healthy and live longer. In a recent study, positive and satisfied middle-aged people were twice as likely to survive over a period of twenty years, as compared to more negative individuals. Optimists have fewer physical and emotional difficulties, experience less pain, enjoy higher energy levels, and are generally happier and calmer. Positive thinking has been found to boost the body's immune system so we can better fight infection. When we feel good, it boosts our self-confidence, which helps us to have better relationships (Essential 3). The MacArthur Study of Successful Aging found that people who are socially connected may survive up to 20 percent longer than those who live more isolated lives. Today, we have many tools to help us connect with others, shore up self-doubt, and make ourselves feel and look younger and more beautiful, both through medical and nonmedical techniques. Despite the myth that libido declines with age, several scientific studies have found that our desire and need for sex continues throughout our lives. A healthy sex life at every age helps lower blood pressure, reduce stress, ward off depression, boost the immune system, diminish pain, maintain physical fitness, and even extend life expectancy.

Stress is among the leading causes of age-related disease (Essential 4). It contributes to physical pain, as well as to the appearance of wrinkles and premature aging. Few people realize that our ability to adapt to our ever-changing environments can greatly contribute to lowering our stress levels. Whether it's traffic, smoke, clutter, noise, mold, smog, or information overload, our quality longevity depends upon our ability to adjust to these environmental influences (Essential 5). Personalizing our immediate surroundings, at home and at work, is an important environmental element that is within our control.

It is much easier to maintain a positive attitude when we enjoy good health, and the best way to ensure that is by eating a healthy diet and staying physically fit. With so many fitness options available, there is bound to be something that appeals to just about everybody. Along with the basics of tennis, jogging, cycling, swimming, and yoga, many people are getting fit with Pilates, weight training, Bosu ball, spinning, salsa dancing, ballet, trail running, and more. Essential 6 will introduce the Longevity Fitness Routine, which covers cardiovascular conditioning, balance and flexibility work, and strength training—the three vital fitness areas for maximizing health, boosting energy levels, and preventing many age-related diseases. Recent research has found that regular physical activity can add two or more years to an individual's life expectancy.

Reducing the clutter in our lives is a powerful way to lower stress levels. Just as it feels good to occasionally clean out your closet and get rid of the clutter there, it can sometimes become necessary to reduce relationship clutter—clean your emotional house—and conserve your energy for the people you love or care about. At times, relationships may become more damaging than they are enriching— old friendships that were once meaningful can become simply old habits that may have negative effects but are hard to break.

A healthy diet can have a major impact on life expectancy by lowering our risk for heart disease, cancer, and other age-related illnesses. Longitudinal studies have found that a diet that emphasizes the right food choices and helps people stay at their target body weight can increase survival rates by 50 percent or more. We'll learn about the Longevity Diet (Essential 7), a healthy diet plan that allows you to eat *all* of your favorite foods—even naughty desserts. It incorporates the best scientific data on healthful eating for longevity and weight control, combined with some of the most satisfying and delicious foods available. Just as fitness experts now tell us that for long-range health, it's best to cross-train our bodies by emphasizing aerobics one day, weight training the next, and perhaps yoga the day after that, the Longevity Diet shows us how to cross-train our eating, allowing us to break free of the boredom and repetition of today's popular low-carbohydrate, South Florida, salmon-every-meal diets.

We can enjoy a barbecued steak and a Caesar salad one day and a delicious pasta dinner with whole-grain crusty bread the next. The Longevity Diet allows our bodies to break free of today's fashionable diets and learn to process all good foods in realistic portions, while feeling sated, satisfied, and anything but deprived.

We will look at the latest in medicines and treatments designed to keep us young (Essential 8). From smart drugs to Botox to microscopic lasers, we'll learn about the options available to keep us looking and feeling youthful throughout our lives. Even simply taking drugs to lower blood pressure has been shown to increase life expectancy by at least two or more years, and scientists have found that cholesterol-lowering statin drugs can increase survival rates of heart patients by more than 50 percent.

Many baby boomers may recall the 1960s Harvard professor who traveled to India and became the guru known as Ram Dass. His "Be here now" message became the mantra for staying in the moment, neither worrying about the past nor stressing over the future. His message echoes that of many other teachers, ranging from Martin Buber to Lao-Tzu.

We don't have to become spiritual gurus to live a long, healthy life, but attempting to stay in the moment helps us to achieve quality longevity. Mindfulness or *mindful awareness*—the subtle process of moment-to-moment awareness of one's thoughts, feelings, and physical states—is key to sharpening memory and staying mentally fit. Initial research suggests that this ability not only reduces stress and anxiety, but also boosts the immune system and promotes health and healing for a variety of medical illnesses and conditions, including heart disease, diabetes, arthritis, and chronic pain.

This underlying principle of mindful awareness can be applied to nearly all of the Eight Essential Strategies. Having an awareness of our bodies and what is going on around us helps us maintain balance and avoid danger. Awareness of our internal sensations reminds us to stop eating when we are sated—a key to maintaining our target body weight. By integrating mindful awareness into our daily lives, we not only enjoy ourselves more and live longer, we take better care of ourselves, have a more positive outlook, and feel more empathy toward others.

Mindfulness often fosters a sense of spirituality, and several studies have found that people who pursue some form of spirituality live longer. Recently, investigators found that visiting a house of worship just once a week can extend life expectancy by nearly a decade. Studies of patients with chronic physical illnesses have found that those who believed in God had a 30 percent lower mortality rate as compared with those who felt abandoned by God. The increased longevity benefits of spirituality result from many of its forms, including religion, meditation, a personal belief in a higher power, and more.

Many of the benefits of *The Longevity Bible*'s Eight Essentials can be achieved in a remarkably short period—as little as fourteen days. My research team at UCLA conducted controlled studies to test how well volunteer subjects could improve their brain and body fitness by focusing on just four of the essential strategies: *mental aerobics, physical fitness, stress management,* and *a healthy diet.*

We found that after just two weeks, the volunteers who followed the healthy longevity lifestyle program (as opposed to the control group who merely continued their usual behavior) experienced improved memory performance and brain efficiency. They also reported greater levels of relaxation and lower levels of stress.

We observed significant physical health benefits as well. Many volunteers on the program lost weight and experienced a significant decline in blood pressure and cholesterol levels.

Shirley I., a thirty-four-year-old social worker raising a young daughter on her own, had always been fastidious and fiercely independent. She lived with a certain level of stress in her life, but it was constant, and she had developed habitual ways to cope. Sometimes she let off steam by shopping. But why not? Imelda Marcos had more than three hundred pairs of shoes and it didn't kill her.

As she had planned, Shirley went back to graduate school and became a licensed psychologist. It was at the outset of her career that she met and began dating a hugely successful investment banker. The attraction was strong and Shirley was falling in love, but she felt he was pressuring her to give up her independence, move in, and get engaged. In time, his sense of humor, intelligence, and "old-fashioned" courting style—flowers, candlelight dinners, Mediterranean cruises—won her over. Eventually she agreed, and they set up a household together with her daughter.

With the added stress of a new career, the pressing needs of a preteen daughter, and the heavy social demands of her fiancé weighing on her, Shirley found herself becoming forgetful for the first time in her life. Little details began falling through the cracks and she actually mixed up a patient's appointment and missed one of her kid's sports events. When her daughter started making jokes about "Mommy losing her memory," Shirley decided to do something about improving her memory and reducing her stress. She came to UCLA and volunteered for our Fourteen-Day Healthy Longevity Study.

After just two weeks on the program, her memory scores improved significantly, she lost three pounds without trying, and felt more relaxed and better able to deal with both her job and her responsibilities at home. Shirley was able to comfort herself with her old, familiar coping styles, and she was happy. So were the shoe departments at Saks and Neiman Marcus.

Shirley's experience was similar to that of many other subjects in the study for whom these essential longevity strategies improved memory and reduced stress, as well as lowered blood pressure and cholesterol levels. Scientific evidence indicates that adopting these lifestyle strategies not only lowers the risk for Alzheimer's disease, but actually increases life expectancy—*making us live longer*—while adding to the quality of those years.

Quality Longevity for the Long Haul

Large-scale, longitudinal aging studies, including the MacArthur Study of Successful Aging, the Baltimore Longitudinal Study of Aging, the Leisure World Cohort Study, and many others, have yielded scientific findings that add to the foundation of *The Longevity Bible's* strategies. The MacArthur Study found that staying connected through social relationships as we get older is linked to longer and better living. A healthy emotional life—founded on intimacy and strong relationships—is associated with a more positive mental state as well as improved physical health and function. Another key finding is that it's almost *never* too late (or too early) to make healthy lifestyle choices and instigate changes to achieve quality longevity.

Whether we are approaching our forties, fifties, sixties, or more, we all face the challenges and rewards of aging. Studies on successful aging have shown that only one third of what predicts how well we age is controlled by genetics. Approximately two thirds is based on our personal lifestyle choices and, therefore, under our own control.

As we learn about the Eight Essentials, we will see how our psychologist, Shirley, and several others tackle the bumps and hurdles that so many of us face as we get older. We will learn how to apply the Eight Essentials, quickly and easily, and begin living a quality longevity lifestyle. If it's true that we're only as young as we feel, then it's time to start feeling, looking, and acting younger today.

Part 2

The Eight Essentials

Essential 1

Sharpen Your Mind

Memory is the mother of all wisdom.

—AESCHYLUS

The newspaper's daily crossword puzzle had long been the high point of Michele R.'s morning routine. Monday's easy puzzle she could do quickly, and in pen. But as the clues got harder throughout the rest of the week, she felt challenged enough to get that "puzzler's high" whenever she could solve them all and complete the puzzle. That all changed when Michele started working the newspaper's new brainteaser—Sudoku. There was nothing easy about it. How could arranging a bunch of numbers in a grid possibly hold her attention for more than a few minutes? Words were so much more interesting than numbers, and she had always been lousy at math.

It only took a week for Michele to get hooked on the new puzzle, as she began to pick up its patterns and logical challenges. She grabbed for the entertainment section of the newspaper before anyone could get near it—Sudoku had become Michele's new obsession. But instead of being fun and challenging like the crossword, it was often frustrating and sometimes enraging. She absolutely couldn't start her day off right if she failed to solve that morning's Sudoku. Her kids joked that if Michele kept up this fixation with the puzzle, she might have to join a Sudoku Anonymous group to kick the habit.

Soon Michele's husband began doing Sudokus as well. They would copy the one in the morning paper and race each other to see who could finish it first. As Michele got better at Sudoku, she began to get that puzzler's high back, and the added excitement of beating her husband every morning made it all the more fun.

Most people enjoy mentally challenging puzzles, especially when they are able to solve them. As Michele did, it's good to find mental challenges and leisure activities that are fun and engaging, but not ones that are so tough that we *strain*, rather than *train* the brain. Staying mentally active sharpens the mind, improves memory, and protects the brain from future decline. This first Essential is the key to following all the Essentials, which empowers us to take control of how we age.

A study published in the *New England Journal of Medicine* found that participating in leisure activities, such as playing board games, reading books, or doing crossword puzzles, cuts the risk for developing Alzheimer's disease by nearly a third. When scientists study animals raised in mentally stimulating cages—those with lots of toys, mazes, and other distractions—the animals not only have an easier time remembering how to navigate their mazes, but their brains' memory centers are much larger than those of animals brought up in standard-issue cages.

Several large-scale studies have found that people who engage in mentally stimulating leisure activities, along with other quality longevity strategies, not only feel happier and function better, but also tend to live longer. The most well-known longitudinal investigation of healthy aging, the MacArthur Study, found that people who remained mentally active—doing puzzles, reading books, playing cards or other games—had better quality of life and longer life expectancy than those who had less mental stimulation.

When scientists compare college-educated volunteers with those who have not attended college, they consistently find a lower risk for Alzheimer's disease among the more educated study volunteers. A recent brain imaging study found that with more years of education, we are better able to use the front part of the brain to augment mental prowess. This is a good argument for continuing education throughout our lifetimes.

The Sharper Mind

According to the scientific evidence, whenever we push ourselves to solve problems in a new way, we may be strengthening the connections between our brain cells. Each brain cell has dendrites. These minute extensions—similar to branches of a tree—pass information along from brain cell to brain cell. Without use, our dendrites can atrophy or shrink; but when we exercise them in new and creative ways, their connections remain active, passing new information along. Basically, any conscious effort to exercise your brain can potentially create new brain cell connections. And, remarkably, new dendrites can still be created even if old ones have already died.

Over the years, we learn more complex mental skills that eventually become automatic, so that our minds can perform certain mental tasks with less effort. As we gain experience, our minds become able to automatically take in the big picture without having to focus on every little detail. Take a look at the following paragraph:

Dont alwyas blveiee what yor'ue rdanieg becusae the hmuan mnid has phaoenmneal pweor. Aoccdrnig to uinervtisy rsceearchers, it deosn't mttaer inwaht odrer the ltteers in a wrod are plcead. Waht is improtnat is taht the frist and lsat letetrs rae in the corerct pclae.

You probably understood the message, yet the delivery was a mess. Our minds have learned to automatically perceive the meaning of something, even if details are missing or wrong. Systematic studies have found that older, healthy people with more experience are better and quicker at assessing an overall scene or picking out a face in a crowd than younger people, who tend to focus on details.

We can fine-tune these skills at any age with mental exercise. To make the most of our brain power and optimize mental sharpness, it is helpful to keep in mind what I call the *P's and Q's for Sharpening the Mind: Presence, Persevere, Quality,* and *Question.*

- *Presence.* Staying focused on the present makes us more efficient in any given mental task. What is key to remaining present and on task is not just the ability to take in what's going on around us, but also being able to shut out what's not important.
- *Persevere.* Sticking with a specific mental task builds learning and memory skills. You may start piano lessons today, but unless you continue to practice over the following weeks and months, you won't gain the mental benefits or the enjoyment of mastering the instrument. With perseverance, your memory skills will improve and you'll enjoy heightened confidence in your cognitive abilities.

- *Quality.* When our minds focus on the qualities, details, and meanings of new information, we retain it longer and have a greater sense of control. This control allows us to organize the information and improves our learning abilities. If our hobbies and leisure activities have qualities that we value, they become more fun and fulfilling. Many people like to get involved in competitions, keeping a prize they value in mind during their activity. This may explain why competitive sports are so exciting for both the participants and the fans.
- *Question.* Curiosity allows us to expand our mental horizons. Reading stimulating books and magazines, exploring unfamiliar places and hobbies, and continually probing and asking questions will keep our mental skills intact.

Applying the *P's* and *Q's* not only helps keep our mental lives active, but it allows us to develop *resilience*, the ability to recover from negative experiences. When we take chances and reasonable risks, explore new opportunities, and learn new skills, we also become better at bouncing back if we should fail in an endeavor. Being able to set and achieve new goals leads to greater self-confidence, personal strength, and a positive outlook (see Essential 2).

Risk-taking and thrill-seeking taken to the extreme are behaviors typical of adolescence, and with maturity most people learn to avoid dangerous activities, thus lengthening their life expectancy. The key is to find a balance—a way to pursue novel experiences that expand the mind without going overboard. The following are a few activities to consider for keeping mentally sharp over the years.

- *Travel.* If your inclination is to head for the beach and plug yourself into a lounge chair during your holidays, consider trying a different kind of vacation, maybe a sightseeing adventure to a destination you've never visited, or perhaps a stay at a self-realization spa or a dude ranch. Many vacation packages and cruises take visitors to new and exotic locations and enrich their experience with informative lectures on the region. Elderhostel (*www.eldershostel.org*) is one of the world's largest educational and travel organizations for people age fifty-five and older.

- *Get creative.* Learning a musical instrument or taking up oil painting are great ways to stimulate the artistic side of the brain, especially if you tend to be an analytical, left-brain type of person. Exploring your talents in right-brain creative pursuits will help keep your brain cells active and possibly protect them from future decline.

- *Challenge yourself.* Take your mental pursuits to the next level. If you do only the easy newspaper crossword puzzles on Mondays and Tuesdays, push yourself and try the more challenging Thursday and Friday puzzles. If you're a whiz at putting together five-hundred-piece jigsaw puzzles, buy a thousand-piece puzzle and get to work.

- *Take on a new hobby.* Whether it's collecting stamps, knitting, climbing rocks, or French cooking, getting involved in a new hobby is a great way to expand the mind. Hobbies distract us from everyday worries and allow us to gain a sense of mastery in whatever area we choose to pursue. People who engage in hobbies are less likely to experience mental decline as they age than those who spend most of their spare time in front of the television.

- *Join a study group or book club.* Some people like to study on their own, while others enjoy the interaction of a group experience. Book clubs and study groups are a popular way to expand your mental horizons and enjoy the company of like-minded learners.

- *Go back to school.* Most colleges and universities have extension classes for part-time students of all ages. Our UCLA Center on Aging has a Senior Scholars Program that makes it easy for older adults to audit undergraduate classes. The intergenerational component of the program enriches the experience for both generations: The undergraduates benefit from the wisdom of their older classmates, who in turn enjoy the youthful energy of returning to a college campus and interacting with a new twenty-something generation.
- *Flex your brain.* Try some Web sites, books, or magazines with puzzles designed to flex your brain muscles. Check out the upcoming mental aerobic exercises, as well as those in the Appendix, which will give you a taste of the range of mental teasers and encourage you to pursue more puzzles. Enjoy some mentally challenging games such as Scrabble or Trivial Pursuit, activities that also can be a fun social event.

Building Brain Mass

A recent study published in the journal *Nature* found that three months of mental training can alter brain structure and, in essence, build brain muscle. After the study volunteers were given MRI brain scans, they were taught to juggle—a mentally challenging task. After three months of juggling, the brain scans were repeated. This time the scans showed significant increases in the volume of gray matter—the outer rim of the brain that is responsible for thinking and complex reasoning. Either their brain cells had grown larger and developed more extensive connections, or the number of brain cells had increased enough to build brain bulk. However, when the volunteers gave up their new hobby, their brains shrank back to their previous sizes. You can build brain muscle but you have to continue your mental activity to sustain the benefits.

In the first study of its kind, our UCLA research team found that when mental aerobics and memory training are combined with other *Longevity Bible* Essential Strategies, not only do volunteers improve their memory abilities but their brains become more efficient. We studied a group of volunteers who had only very mild age-related memory complaints—the kinds of occasional slips typical of people in their forties and fifties: walking into a room and forgetting the reason why, or having trouble recalling a word without a delay. Half of the group spent about twenty minutes each day on a mental aerobics program—learning memory techniques and solving puzzles—and kept physically active and ate a healthy diet. The other half of the study volunteers served as a control group and did not make any lifestyle changes during the two-week period. All volunteers received PET scans to measure their brain activity before and after the study.

Those who followed the healthy longevity lifestyle program had a highly significant change in brain efficiency in a region in the front part of the brain that controls everyday memory tasks, or "working memory." Working memory allows people to keep a limited amount of information in their minds for a brief period—such as when you get a phone number from Directory Assistance and remember it just long enough to dial it.

Just as athletes build physical stamina and muscular efficiency when they work out with a trainer at the gym, the healthy-lifestyle volunteers appeared to be building more efficient "brain muscle." Our study results suggested that focused mental activity and memory training can lead to greater brain efficiency—those on the program needed to use *less* brain energy to perform *better* on mental tasks.

For some study volunteers, this effect was dramatic. Michele R., a forty-six-year-old retired pharmacist and mother of three school children, admitted to having too many responsibilities on her plate. She was constantly carpooling, volunteering, and attempting to keep up with her endless list of chores and errands. Before entering the healthy longevity research study, she had begun to notice her memory slips, particularly when she was under pressure or multi-tasking. Her memory test scores showed that her verbal memory was typical for a woman of her age—not quite as good as it was when she was in college or pharmacy school, but about average for her age group. When we performed a brain stress test—a functional MRI scan that monitored activity during a memory task—the scanner showed a large area of the brain working hard while she performed the memory tasks.

After practicing *The Longevity Bible*'s memory techniques and spending time exercising her brain with mental aerobics each day, the brain stress tests showed that she needed to use very little of her brain's memory centers to successfully recall new information, and her verbal memory scores had increased by 200 percent—a dramatic improvement that made her memory more typical of a twenty-five-year-old than of a forty-six-year-old. With just two weeks of practice, Michele had subtracted more than twenty years from her brain age.

Memory Training 101

Memory defines who we are, now and at every moment. It also defines our future, because without memory ability, we cannot make plans and think ahead. And, of course, without memory, it's as if we have no past. Staying mentally sharp requires optimum memory performance, the foundation for any quality longevity program.

On Nancy G.'s fortieth birthday, she came home from work to find her husband's gift: a beautifully typed divorce petition. Unable to discuss the divorce rationally with her own mother, who was in the early stages of Alzheimer's disease, Nancy was forced to spend the ensuing years nursing her mother as well as her two teenage daughters through the trauma of Daddy going to live with his new, pretty "friend." Because she had to bump her part-time marketing job up to full-time, Nancy gave up her yoga classes and morning hikes with friends.

Nancy was already too busy or exhausted to read her novels or do the crossword puzzle at night, and it now seemed like the girls needed hours of help with their studies. Nancy's mother's health was declining daily, and Nancy's boss was insisting that she begin traveling for work. And though she finally met someone she was interested in dating, even that was causing tension because he was constantly asking for more time alone with her.

Nancy began getting stress headaches like those she'd had in college. But what really worried her was how forgetful she was becoming—a client's name here, an appointment there, mixing up one of the girls' teacher conferences with another school function, and so on. Nancy had always prided herself on being responsible and prompt, and now she was panicked—was she getting Alzheimer's disease like her mother?

When Nancy came to UCLA seeking help, she learned about *The Longevity Bible* Essential Strategies. She almost immediately improved her memory abilities using simple techniques like *Look, Snap, Connect*, along with some other, more advanced memory techniques. Nancy came to understand that genetics accounts for only one third of what predicts whether or not someone will get Alzheimer's disease. She learned that she could stave off and possibly prevent symptoms even if it turned out she was genetically at risk. She began to feel more empowered, which sharply lowered her stress levels. The reduction of Nancy's anxiety levels not only helped improve her memory, it relieved her headaches and gave her more energy for all aspects of her life.

The memory techniques that I taught Nancy are simple and easy to learn. Whether you need to remember a shopping list, the name and face of a new acquaintance, or the heights of the ten tallest buildings in the world, you can accomplish any of those tasks with my three basic memory techniques: *Look, Snap, Connect.*

Look reminds us to focus our attention. The most common explanation for memory loss is that the information never gets into our minds in the first place, usually because we are distracted or multitasking. Reminding ourselves to focus our attention will dramatically boost our memory power.

Snap stands for creating a mental snapshot or visual image — in our mind's eye — of the information to be remembered. For most people, visual images are much easier to remember than other forms of information.

Connect means we need to link up the visual images in a meaningful way. These associations are the key to drumming up memories when we want to recall them later.

Getting interested in what you are trying to learn and infusing the information with personal meaning will make these techniques more effective. Experiments with expert chess players have shown that they can readily memorize the chess pieces on the board if the pieces are placed as they would be during a match, but the players' ability to recall a pattern of pieces placed at random is almost impossible. One arrangement of chess pieces has meaning, while the other does not.

If I were to briefly introduce you to my friend Sylvia at a crowded party, it is quite possible you would forget her name. However, if you were to mention that she reminds you of your college roommate who also happened to be named Sylvia—giving my friend's name personal meaning for you—you would probably always remember my friend Sylvia's name.

When linking up your mental snapshots, create a story that has action and detail. If a picture is worth a thousand words, then a Technicolor motion picture is probably worth a million. Try memorizing the following eight words using Look, Snap, Connect. Create eight visual images and link them together in a story.

> Whistle
> Grandmother
> Sweater
> Juggler
> Cherries
> Ping-Pong
> Poodles
> Bow tie

Spend a moment coming up with a story before reading on.

Almost everyone's story will come out differently. If you like ridiculous stories, as I do, then you might be imagining a grandmother blowing a whistle as she knits a sweater. She gives the sweater to her grandson, who is juggling three cherries. One of the cherries gets away from him and interrupts his poodles' Ping-Pong game. Look closely, because the poodles have on bright red bow ties.

Notice my story's detail, action, and attempt at humor. All these elements make it easier for me to learn the words and recall them later. If you prefer more logical stories, then you might have the juggler wear the bow tie and let the grandmother eat the cherries. This technique works well for remembering everyday memory tasks and errands such as grocery lists or picking up a package at the post office after work.

Name That Face

Nancy G.'s memory complaints included difficulty with names and faces, and she is not alone: That is the most common form of forgetfulness as we age. Nancy was able to improve her ability to recall a person's name after recognizing his or her face by applying a variation of Look, Snap, Connect.

Whenever she met someone whose name she wanted to remember, she imagined a *Name Snap* (visual image reminding her of the person's name) and a *Face Snap* (a distinguishing facial or other body feature), and then used Connect to link the two Snaps together. When she met new coworker Lucille, she noticed her bright red hair (Face Snap), which reminded her of Lucille Ball (Name Snap). To connect these two Snaps, Nancy imagined Lucille Ball working in the next cubicle over, where the new Lucille would now be working.

Some names automatically trigger a visual image—meet Mrs. Taylor and you can picture her sewing a dress. Mr. Baker could be checking on his cake. Ms. Hill might be standing on top of a knoll. Other names evoke the image of a famous individual with the same name. You may visualize Mr. Fields on his tractor or eating his wife's chocolate chip cookies.

Not all names readily lend themselves to mental snapshots, so you may need to substitute visually evocative words that sound like or rhyme with the name. For Ms. Balisok, perhaps you see a ball of socks. When you meet Mr. Haft, you might see him floating on half a raft.

Try to come up with a visual image for each of the following names so you can create a Name Snap:

> Herzog
>
> Gambhir
>
> Potvin

There is no right answer, but you could imagine seeing Mrs. Herzog driving a hearse with a hog as a passenger. Perhaps Mr. Gambhir is playing a Monopoly game while drinking a beer, and Ms. Potvin may have landscaped her yard with pots full of growing vines.

Memory Masters Reveal Their Tricks

For some motivated individuals, their memory feats become a competitive sport. These memory mavens challenge each other at international contests and manage to memorize remarkably large numbers and amounts of trivia.

Scientists at University College London found that these master memorizers are not that different from the rest of us. Their IQs are not extraordinary and their brain structures are unremarkable. What they do share are the strategies for accomplishing these memory feats, as well as the way their brains function when performing these mental tasks. The memory strategies activate a network of brain regions known to be involved in spatial navigation and memory.

One of the most commonly used memory techniques is called the Roman Room Method, wherein you visualize yourself walking through a familiar route, such as a sequence of rooms in your home, and mentally place images of the items to be remembered at specific points on the route. When you want to recall the items, you simply retrace your steps. This strategy has been around since ancient Roman orators used it to help them recall the specifics of their speeches.

We all can become memory masters by learning this technique. Start with your apartment or house and take a mental walk through the rooms. In each room, mentally deposit an object you want to remember, such as your blue suit hanging on the back of the front door, ready to go to the tailor's, or your phone book on the bathroom counter, open to the number of your dentist, whom you need to call for an appointment. Before long, your routes can include your office, your sister's beach house, and so on, until you have committed to memory more information than you ever wanted to know. I may have to name my next book *How to Forget What You Don't Want to Remember* in order to help some people reset their overstuffed memory storage units.

It's Never Too Late to Boost Memory Power

Nancy's mother was already suffering from the early stages of Alzheimer's disease. She had shown some improvement after treatment with Aricept and Namenda (see Essential 8), but even with the medicine, Nancy's mom was not the same woman she had been just a few years earlier. Nancy had heard that some of the mental exercises that she herself had been practicing could be simplified so that her mother would find them stimulating and not too challenging.

Recent studies suggest that people who have early stage Alzheimer's disease may be capable of learning more than previously thought. Dr. David Loewenstein and associates at Mount Sinai Medical Center in Miami Beach, Florida, taught Alzheimer's patients memory skills to improve name and face recognition over a three-month period. They found that the intervention improved recall of faces and names by 170 percent, and the improvement was sustained over the following three-month period. In another study of Alzheimer's patients, an eight-week mental stimulation program, in combination with the antidementia medicine Aricept, significantly improved patient interactions and overall functioning levels.

Mental Aerobics

Whether you are a puzzle fanatic or just a beginner, I've included some mental aerobic exercises to get you started and help you to advance to the next level of challenge. Keeping the mind active and alert is an essential component of any comprehensive quality longevity program, so start out at the level you think matches your needs, whether it's beginning, intermediate, or advanced.

Brain teasers and puzzles often involve *lateral thinking*, which means that we are trying to solve a problem from many angles instead of tackling it head on. When you get stumped with a puzzle, try thinking "outside the box"—see if you can come up with a new and creative solution. When you do, you'll not only be fortifying your brain cells, you'll probably experience a sense of intellectual gratification.

It's also a good idea to cross-train your brain. For right-handed people, the right side, or hemisphere, of the brain controls spatial relationships and the left side specializes in verbal skills and logical analysis. I've labeled most of the puzzles according to the hemisphere that tends to work the hardest when you're searching for the solution. Cross-train by exercising both sides of the brain.

You'll find the answers to the exercises at the end of each section. If you come up with an alternative answer, be sure to let me know at *www.DrGarySmall.com*.

Beginning Exercises

1. *Warm-up Exercise.* Brush your hair using your nondominant hand (i.e., if you're right-handed, use your left hand). You'll notice that it is awkward at first, but practice this exercise over the next few days and you'll see how much easier it gets.

2. *Beginner's Number-Placement Puzzle.* Fill in the grid so that every row, every column, and every two-by-two box contains the digits 1 through 4.

1	2	3	4
4	3	1	2
2	1	4	3
3	4	2	1

3. *Whole-Brain Exercise.* Say "silk" six times. What do cows drink?

4. *Left-Brain Exercise.* See how many words you can spell from the letters below. No letter may be used twice, and each word must contain the letter *L*.

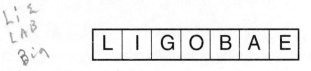

L	I	G	O	B	A	E

5. *Left-Brain Exercise.* How many months have twenty-eight days?

6. *Left-Brain Exercise.* All of the vowels have been removed from the following proverb, and the remaining consonants are in the correct sequence, broken up into groups of two to five letters. Replace the vowels and figure out the proverb.

STRK   WHLTH   RNS   HT

7. *Right-Brain Exercise.* Figure out which object does not match the others.

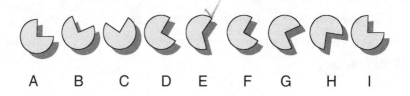

A   B   C   D   E   F   G   H   I

8. *Whole-Brain Exercise.* Figure out the word suggested by the message below.

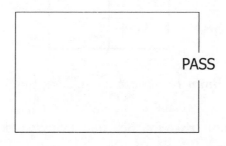

PASS

Answers to Beginning Exercises

1. *Warm-up Exercise.* No right answer.
2. *Beginner's Number-Placement Puzzle.*

1	2	3	4
4	3	1	2
2	1	4	3
3	4	2	1

OR

1	2	4	3
4	3	1	2
2	1	3	4
3	4	2	1

3. *Whole-Brain Exercise.* Cows generally drink water, unless they are like me and sometimes prefer sparkling water. If you said "milk," then you might need to slow down a bit and focus your attention.

4. *Left-Brain Exercise.* I came up with the following words: AGILE, AIL, ALE, BAGEL, BAIL, BALE, BLOG, BOIL, EL, GAIL, GALE, GEL, GLIB, GLOB, GLOBE, GOAL, GOALIE, LAB, LAG, LEA, LEG, LEGO, LIB, LIE, LOB, LOBE, LOG, LOGE, OBLIGE

5. *Whole-Brain Exercise.* All of them.

6. *Left-Brain Exercise.* STRIKE WHILE THE IRON IS HOT.

7. *Right-Brain Exercise.* E (the angle is wider than that in all the other figures).

8. *Whole-Brain Exercise.* PASS THROUGH.

Once you feel you have mastered the above exercises, continue to aerobicize your brain by moving on to the more challenging exercises below.

Intermediate Exercises

1. *Warm-up Exercise.* Sit down at the computer and try using the mouse with your nondominant hand. Browse the Internet and see how well you do. This is an excellent exercise for anyone suffering from tendonitis due to mouse overuse. Practice over the next few days to see if you can improve your skills.

2. *Letter-Placement Puzzle.* Now we're going to substitute letters for the numbers, to make it slightly tougher. Fill in the grid so that every row, every column, and every two-by-two box contains the letters A, B, C, and D.

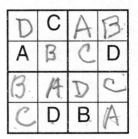

3. *Left-Brain Exercise.* See how many words you can spell from the letters below. No letter may be used twice, and each word must contain the letter "M."

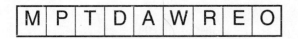

4. *Right-Brain Exercise.* The following arrangement of sticks forms six squares. Try to remove four sticks so that the remaining unmoved sticks form two rectangles.

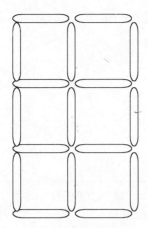

5. *Left-Brain Exercise*. Starting with the word WARM, change one letter at a time until you have the word FILE. Each change must result in a proper word.

WARM

FARM

FARE

FIRE

FILE

6. *Whole-Brain Exercise*. Count up the number of *F*'s in the following sentence.

FRESH FISH IS AN EXCELLENT SOURCE OF OMEGA-3 AND A BETTER SOURCE OF ANTIOXIDANTS THAN MANY REALIZE. *2*

7. *Right-Brain Exercise*. By making just one move in a single direction, see if you can make all the sticks form a triangle.

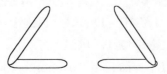

8. *Whole-Brain Exercise.* Figure out the word suggested by the message below.

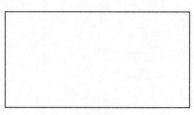

COVER

Answers to Intermediate Exercises

1. *Warm-up Exercise.* No right answer.
2. *Letter-Placement Puzzle.*

D	C	A	B
A	B	C	D
B	A	D	C
C	D	B	A

3. *Left-Brain Exercise.* Here are some of the words I found: ADMIRE, AM, DAM, DORM, DRAM, DREAM, DREAMT, EM, MA, MAD, MADE, MAP, MAR, MARE, MART, MAT, MATE, MATED, MEAT, MET, MEW, MOP, MOPED, MORE, MOW, MOWER, PRAM, RAMP, RAM, ROAM, ROME, ROMP, TAME, TAMED, TAMP, TEAM, TEMPT, TERM, TRAM, WAM, WARM, WARMED, WORM

4. *Right-Brain Exercise.* The solution below contains a smaller rectangle within a larger one.

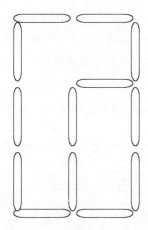

5. *Left-Brain Exercise.* WARM, FARM, FIRM, FILM, FILE, or WARM, FARM, FIRM, FIRE, FILE.

6. *Whole-Brain Exercise.* Many people count two, but the correct answer is four. Our brains often just don't process the word "of."

7. *Right-Brain Exercise.* If you slowly bring the page closer to your face, you will see an image of a triangle.

8. *Whole-Brain Exercise.* UNDERCOVER

Now take a two-minute stress-release break and breathe deeply and slowly, so you will be prepared for the brain-busters below.

Advanced Exercises

1. *Warm-up Exercise.* See if you can draw the three-dimensional figure below, using your nondominant hand:

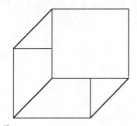

2. Advanced Number-Placement Puzzle. Now we're going to make it tougher by jumping from four to six numbers. Fill in the grid so that every row, every column, and every three-by-two box contains the digits 1 through 6. Unless you are an off-the-charts genius or an idiot savant, you will need a pencil with an eraser.

1	4	2	6	3	5
6	5	3	4	1	2
2	6	4	3	5	1
3	1	5	2	4	6
4	3	6	1	2	5
5	2	1	4	6	3

3. Whole-Brain Exercise. Add two lines to complete the sequence below.

4. Left-Brain Exercise. Which is the odd one out?
GROUPER CATFISH PUFFER ANGELFISH

5. ***Whole-Brain Exercise.*** Figure out the message suggested below.

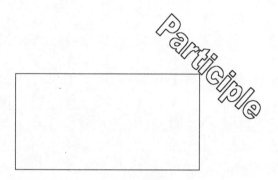

6. ***Left-Brain Exercise.*** How many triangles of any size are in the figure?

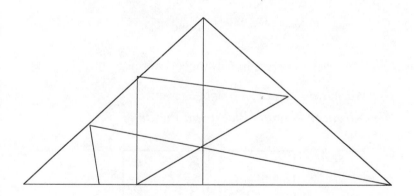

7. ***Whole-Brain Exercise.*** A truck that is one hundred feet long is moving one hundred feet per minute. It must cross a bridge that is one hundred feet in length. How long does it take the truck to cross the bridge?

8. ***Mental Aerobics Word Finder.*** Find and circle the words in the grid on the next page, which appear forward, backward, up, down, and diagonally.

P	O	H	S	I	F	E	S	A	C	N
F	O	D	D	O	O	F	O	R	I	O
O	S	N	O	F	R	O	M	A	N	W
C	O	O	Y	Z	G	E	E	S	O	H
I	A	X	T	E	E	B	G	A	M	E
B	R	A	I	N	T	E	A	S	E	R
O	E	R	E	D	I	B	T	O	N	E
R	L	L	A	C	E	R	H	O	M	E
E	A	U	X	T	E	A	R	E	E	D
A	X	O	T	S	A	C	E	N	T	I
B	A	S	S	N	E	V	E	R	I	R

Axon	Foci	Nowhere	Relax
Bass	Forget	Omega three	Roman
Brainteaser	Game	Oxide	Stress
Doze	Mnemonic	Recall	
Fish	Never	Reed	

Answers to Advanced Exercises

1. **Warm-up Exercise.** No right answer.
2. **Advanced Number-Placement Puzzle.**

1	3	2	6	5	4
4	5	6	3	1	2
2	6	4	5	3	1
3	1	5	2	4	6
6	4	3	1	2	5
5	2	1	4	6	3

3. **Whole-Brain Exercise.** Create an "X" with the two lines to complete the inverted letter sequence.

$\bigwedge \bigvee \bigwedge \bigwedge \sqcap \perp$

4. **Left-Brain Exercise.** CATFISH is the only freshwater fish. All the others are saltwater fish.

5. **Whole-Brain Exercise.** Dangling participle.

6. **Left-Brain Exercise.** Twenty-four.

7. **Whole-Brain Exercise.** Two minutes. During the first minute, the front of the truck will cross the bridge, and during the second minute, the rest of the truck will cross it.

8. **Mental Aerobics Word Finder.**

P	O	H	S	I	F	E	S	A	C	N
F	O	D	D	O	O	F	O	R	I	O
O	S	N	O	F	R	O	M	A	N	W
C	O	O	Y	Z	G	E	E	S	O	H
L	A	X	T	E	E	B	G	A	M	E
B	R	A	I	N	T	E	A	S	E	R
O	E	R	E	D	I	B	T	O	N	E
R	L	L	A	C	E	R	H	O	M	E
E	A	U	X	T	E	A	R	E	E	D
A	X	O	T	S	A	C	E	N	T	I
B	A	S	S	N	E	V	E	R	I	R

For extra credit, see if you can find these other words

Beet	Even	Omen	Sore	Vat
Bide	Foe	Pony	Soul	Yet
Bore	Food	Red	Tear	Zen
Carb	Home	Ride	Tease	
Cast	Item	Shop	Tie	
Cent	Lace	Soar	Tone	

Keeping Your Mind Sharp

- To get the most out of your mental workouts, apply the *P*'s and *Q*'s for Sharpening the Mind: 1) maintain *presence* and focus; 2) *persevere* in your endeavors to further sharpen your mind; 3) look for the *quality* and meaning in things; and 4) always *question* to learn more.
- Try a different approach to expanding your mental horizons, whether it's traveling to new destinations, learning a musical instrument, taking up ballroom dancing, or going back to school.
- Learn and use the three basic memory techniques:
  - –Look: Focus attention on what you want to remember.
  - –Snap: Imagine a mental snapshot of the information.
  - –Connect: Link the snapshots together in your mind's eye.
- Practice other memory strategies for remembering names and faces.
- Stay mentally active through puzzles, games, reading, and other stimulating hobbies, but be sure to train and not strain your brain—find the level of challenge that keeps you interested without frustrating or exhausting you.

Essential 2

Keep a Positive Outlook

A positive attitude may not solve all your problems,
but it will annoy enough people to make it worth the effort.

— HERM ALBRIGHT

You're throwing a dinner party for the new boss and his wife, and everyone from the office is coming. You nabbed the best caterer in town, your house is spotless, and your wife looks fantastic. The bartender is the only staff that's arrived so far, and he's handing out cocktails to the earliest guests. But where the hell is the caterer? Your wife tells you not to worry—he'll get there any minute.

An hour later, the party is hopping and the boss is laughing, but you are freaking out because you just learned that the caterer's truck broke down and the food may not arrive for another two hours. Your wife hands you a drink and tells you to relax, she's got it completely under control.

Your wife walks calmly into the kitchen, wondering "What the X#@!?$* am I going to do now?!" The boss's wife follows her in and says she overheard the whole thing and wants a peek at the pantry. They pull out several boxes of linguini, grab some fresh garlic, butter, and frozen shrimp. Two other women join them and start chopping tomatoes for bruschetta, which they start blowing out of there on crackers as hors d'oeuvres. The bartender brings them a bottle of wine and a few glasses, and suddenly it's a cooking party in the kitchen.

Later, you're eating this pasta your wife threw together, the boss is making toasts to his hosts, everybody *seems* to be having a great time, but *you* know they're all just faking it in a futile attempt not to hurt your feelings over this giant bomb of a dinner party. That caterer is toast.

On Monday, you slink into the office, avoiding all eye contact, especially with the boss—you may have to say good-bye to your corner office after that party fiasco. But the boss follows you down the hall and throws his arm around you. "What an evening! And your wife is incredible! The food was amazing." You look at him dumbfounded. He goes on effusively. "I really admire you—you're a guy who can make the most of a tough situation—like when a caterer blows you off when the new boss is coming over! I love it! I know you're going to move up in this company."

Here's a cheerful thought: Science shows that keeping a positive attitude helps us stay healthy and live longer. A recent Mayo Clinic study found that individuals scoring high in optimism on the MMPI (Minnesota Multiphasic Personality Inventory) were 50 percent more likely to survive the next thirty years than pessimists were. These optimists also had fewer physical and emotional difficulties, were less limited by pain, enjoyed higher energy levels, and were generally happier and calmer.

Everyday stressors from work, family, health issues, social commitments, and countless other challenges can make it tough to stay upbeat, and many factors contribute to whether one has a tendency toward optimism or pessimism. Genes play a role, but so do our early childhood experiences, family background, self-esteem, and degree of spirituality—all of these influences affect our ability to think in a positive way. However, in the pursuit of quality longevity, it is possible to train ourselves to see the cup half *full* instead of half empty. Maintaining a positive attitude, like any other skill, can be learned.

Optimists Win the Longevity Game

Positive thinkers tend to avoid depression, which is known to shorten one's lifespan, especially when not adequately treated. Optimists are also more likely to get timely medical help because they anticipate that they can improve or prevent their health problems. Researchers at Aarhus University Hospital in Denmark considered another possible mechanism for the connection between positive thinking and health—the immune system, the body's means for fighting off infection. In looking at more than three hundred volunteers between the ages of seventy and eighty-five, they found that those who continually ruminated on negative thoughts had higher counts of white blood cells, as if their bodies were trying to fight off a disease. This suggests that negativity may have an adverse effect on health by actually stimulating a physiological response.

People with a prevailing positive outlook are also more inclined to feel content with their lives, and self-satisfaction has been associated with longer life expectancy. Scientists in Finland studied the impact of a sense of well-being and happiness on longevity and found that satisfied people were twice as likely to survive after twenty years compared with individuals who claimed to be dissatisfied.

Those of us who have a generally positive attitude toward aging live longer than those who do not. Dr. Becca Levy and her associates at Yale University explored the influence of attitude on life expectancy in a study that followed over seven hundred individuals for more than two decades. They found that older people who viewed aging in a positive light lived seven and a half years longer than those who saw aging as a more negative experience. If you anticipate a vital, healthy, and fulfilling future, that perception may indeed come true.

In Pursuit of Happiness

Some scientists believe that our brains may be hardwired in ways that determine how happy we tend to be. Dr. Richard Davidson and his colleagues at the University of Wisconsin have pinpointed an area in the front part of the brain that controls positive feelings, optimism, and happiness. His group studied one of the most powerful positive sets of emotions—a mother's feelings toward her newborn baby. Using functional MRI brain scans, they found that when mothers viewed photos of their babies, their brain activity increased dramatically in this front brain region, as compared with the brain activity of mothers viewing photos of unfamiliar infants.

Research also shows that joyful individuals share certain personality traits and habits. For generally upbeat people, happiness is associated with a personality type that emphasizes independence, self-esteem, competence, and close relationships.

Fortunately, even if there is some hardwiring that predisposes us to joy, much of what determines our happiness is under our own control. Although some people pursue it through fancy vacations, expensive cars, jewelry, or other material things, the thrill of these quick-fix gratifications is generally short-lived. Sustained contentment is more likely to result from healthy relationships and meaningful accomplishments.

Ironically, a tragedy or loss can sometimes set individuals on a path to sustained happiness. Many people who survived the 9/11 disaster but were close enough to experience the destruction firsthand were initially devastated, but they eventually got a clearer perspective on what is truly important in their lives—family, friends, and sustaining a purpose in life. Through adversity, people often become more aware of their own survival skills, resilience, emotional strength, and power to help others as well as to be helped. Nobody's life is free of misfortune, but through adversity we can become more aware of little things we often forget to appreciate, and sometimes gain new positive perspectives and insights for the future.

Dr. Ronnie Janoff-Bulman and colleagues at the University of Massachusetts have studied the way profound life events—both positive and negative—may influence an individual's ability to enjoy *sustained* happiness and fulfillment. They compared the well-being of two groups: lottery winners and people who had suddenly become paralyzed. Though the lottery winners experienced initial euphoria following their new wealth, in the long run many were no happier than the accident victims, in part because normal, everyday pleasures now paled next to the thrill of winning the "big one." In contrast, many of the people who became paralyzed learned to adjust to their new disabilities, and were eventually better able to appreciate small pleasures and accomplishments, as compared with the nouveau riche in the study.

Longevity Through Spirituality

Throughout history, various forms of spirituality and religion have been a way for people to embrace a more positive outlook and find deeper meaning in life. Although organized religion is a major influence in many people's lives throughout the world, spirituality is a broad concept and isn't necessarily connected to a specific belief system or form of worship. Some people satisfy their spiritual needs though meditation, music, or art, while others seek harmony with nature or the universe. Whatever form your spiritual expression takes, it can not only help you to feel more secure and manage your stress, but can also extend your life expectancy.

Several scientific studies have found that regular church attendance is associated with longer life. One recent study showed that visiting a house of worship just once each week extends average life expectancy by seven years. The scientists found that this church-going/longevity connection held up even when they factored out the influences of the social support and healthy lifestyles associated with organized religion.

Some people believe that their faith in a higher power keeps them healthy and heals their illnesses. Dr. Kenneth Pargament and his associates at Bowling Green State University in Ohio studied nearly six hundred medical patients and found that those who believed in God had a 30 percent lower mortality rate as compared with those who felt abandoned by God. However, not all studies demonstrate a connection between faith and health. For example, faith has not been found to improve recovery from serious injuries or acute illnesses, or slow the growth of cancer cells. But faith seems to help people face their injury or illness in a way that nurtures acceptance of their human frailty.

Although scientific studies have not definitively confirmed that faith heals, when faced with crises or illnesses beyond their control, many people find that prayer helps them cope, and research points to other health benefits as well. Dr. Harold Koenig and colleagues at Duke University interviewed over eight hundred medical inpatients and found that those embracing religious beliefs or some type of spirituality had better social support, less depression, and higher cognitive function.

The chanting and prayer that is typical of organized religions share many of the mental and physiological qualities of meditation, and scientists have pointed to studies on meditation to explain how faith and religion may help heal our bodies. Research has demonstrated that meditation can positively modify brain activity, immune function, and the body's stress response, as well as lower heart rate and blood pressure. It can also help people achieve a state of mindful awareness, allowing them to stay more present and attuned to what is going on around them. This often leads to a more positive outlook, particularly for people who are easily distracted or habitually multitasking.

Mainstream medicine is recognizing the importance of the interaction between spirituality and health. Neuroscientists have been able to pinpoint specific areas of the brain that are activated when people pray. The meditative state typical of intense prayer has been found to lower blood pressure and heart rate, which reduces the body's stress response (see Essential 4). Nearly two out of every three U.S. medical schools now offer courses on spirituality. Some medical students actually follow the hospital chaplains on their rounds to learn firsthand how the clergy help people who are suffering from physical illnesses.

Confidence—the Longevity Benefits

Having a positive attitude often leads to increased self-confidence, because with a positive attitude we are more likely to believe that we can solve problems and exert control over our environment and ourselves. In the MacArthur Study, investigators found that study volunteers who rated high in self-confidence were more likely to believe that they could improve and maintain their memory skills. Self-confidence was also associated with better physical performance and a greater sense of empowerment. Older people who were able to meet challenges and solve problems had a much better sense of their abilities to live independently, regardless of their actual abilities. These positive self-perceptions greatly improved their quality of life.

Self-confidence and self-esteem are character traits that form early in our development. Our sense of self is often influenced by our childhood experiences. At a young age, we begin to compare ourselves to others. One might have been stronger, taller, cuter, or smarter than one's playmates in the sandbox, but those playmates might have had more doting grandparents or better handball skills or longer curls. This kind of competitive comparison of our own attributes to those of others can either bolster or deflate our self-esteem. An abusive parent or even a negative comment at the wrong time or place can erode our confidence, whereas our early successes or encouragement from parents can positively shape our future self-perceptions.

Self-esteem affects almost every aspect of life. When we feel good about ourselves, we have more fulfilling relationships, we're more resilient, we feel more upbeat and are better able to cope with adversity. Unfortunately, too often people focus much of their self-esteem on physical appearance and the attainment of wealth rather than on values, personality traits, integrity, and behavior. Certainly, living a quality longevity lifestyle—eating healthfully, limiting stress, and staying fit—helps people not only to feel younger, but to look younger as well.

But it is sometimes hard to live up to the perfect, youth-obsessed images constantly bombarding us in magazines, television, and films. This becomes an increasing challenge as we age. Although no one can stop time, with the latest preventive measures and modern medical treatments, we *can* take years off our appearance (see Essential 8). Older people sometimes complain of feeling invisible or overlooked, as if they are "fading into the background." The sooner a person can shake off the desire to conform to an idealized, unrealistic, and usually unattainable "supermodel/super-wealthy image," the healthier they will be physically and emotionally, and the greater their self-esteem.

Building Self-Esteem

Anyone who has ever experienced a period of low self-esteem knows it can certainly fuel a negative outlook. Some simple exercises can help provide a positive spin and clearer perspective on negative perceptions one might have about oneself.

DOING THE RIGHT THING

Matching your actions to your beliefs is a great self-esteem builder. As much as possible, make choices and act in ways that fit with your beliefs about moral behavior. Perform a small act of kindness to a stranger or to someone you care about, make a charitable donation, or perhaps pledge your time for a good cause. Helping others and supporting causes one believes in usually makes people feel good about themselves.

INNER CRITIC AND REBUTTAL EXERCISE

The following chart has two columns, Inner Critic and Rebuttals. Under Inner Critic, write down three examples of ways in which you might criticize yourself. Next to each criticism, list several rebuttals. For example, you might write that you're not very good at your job because you didn't get a promotion and you haven't been giving it your all lately. In the rebuttal column, you can dispute this negative perception by listing your professional achievements; things you enjoy about your job; and recognition you may have received from your boss or coworkers in the past. You may find that your critical belief is a distortion when you recall your work achievements, the aspects of your job that you really like, and how much your coworkers respect you.

Inner Critic and Rebuttal Exercise

In the left-hand column below, list three examples of negative self-perceptions, then rebut each of them in the right-hand column.

Inner Critic	Rebuttals
1. _____	1. _____
	_____
	_____
2. _____	2. _____
	_____
	_____
3. _____	3. _____
	_____
	_____

Drinking from the Half-Full Cup

Some people get more wrapped up in sadness, worry, and negative thoughts than others. By always anticipating the worst, some of these individuals don't just worry about possible future disappointments—they practically guarantee them. If individuals believe that even their best efforts will not lead to achieving their goals, they rarely take risks or invest all their energy in their endeavors; hence, they essentially undercut their own chances at success.

Over time, embracing negative thoughts and feelings can lead to depression. Psychotherapy, medication, or both can often help, and for most of us depression is just a temporary bump that may follow a disappointment, missed opportunity, or failed attempt. However, when some people get depressed, they can fall into a rut of negative thinking. They may retreat from the outside world and anticipate only failure and disappointment around every corner. They can lose interest in family, friends, hobbies, and jobs, and for these individuals professional treatment is firmly recommended.

Jim S., fifty-seven, a successful trial attorney, was respected by his colleagues and well known for his high-profile celebrity cases. Although he truly enjoyed helping his clients when they needed him the most, his "day job" was getting a little bit dull. Jim had always liked new challenges, and he was searching for a way to be more creative. After being asked to write a couple of articles for a trade journal, Jim found he really got a creative charge out of it. And it was much more fun than the tedious legalese of his case material. When he met a literary agent at a dinner party, she encouraged Jim to consider writing a proposal for a book featuring some of his most noteworthy trials.

Jim was pumped up about the book proposal and started working on it every night. He had fantasies of taking time off from the firm and launching a literary career—maybe he would try a mystery novel after his first book hit the best-seller list. After all, John Grisham started out as a lawyer—and his books even became movies! The more Jim got into the book proposal, the less he enjoyed going to work at his law firm.

Jim finally turned in his proposal and anxiously waited for the agent's response. When she called, she was enthusiastic about it and sent the proposal out to over a dozen New York editors. Jim could already see himself doing a national book tour, appearing on the morning talk shows, and having gala book-signings. Maybe he would give up trial law altogether—he certainly wouldn't miss the pressure and the long hours.

Although a couple of editors expressed some initial interest in his proposal, no solid offers came in; just rejection letters saying there were already too many books out on the same topic. One editor suggested that if the cases in Jim's book focused on political figures, there might be some interest, since a major election was coming up next year. Jim's agent encouraged him to rewrite the proposal with this political spin.

Jim initially agreed, but every time he sat down to do the rewrite, he felt overwhelmed and frustrated. He was a harsh critic—as soon as he put something down on paper, he'd reread it and cross it out. The "charge" he'd gotten from writing the proposal was gone, and it had become a daunting endeavor. He couldn't keep his mind on it and kept procrastinating. He finally admitted to himself that he was never going to write the thing.

Jim felt humiliated for getting carried away with his fantasies of literary fame. He'd become distracted from his job as a trial lawyer, and even though he tried to throw himself back into it, that work now seemed even duller than before.

Worst of all, Jim had lost his confidence—not just in writing, but in his law practice as well. If his chance of becoming a famous author could vanish so quickly, maybe he would lose the next case, too. Soon his pessimism was tainting everything he did—if his wife planned a picnic on the weekend, he would ruminate about rain. If he had a meeting across town, Jim fretted that the traffic would make him late. He felt anxious and easily agitated, and he wasn't sleeping well. Jim's wife grew concerned that he was becoming depressed and pressed him to seek professional help.

After a couple of months of psychotherapy, Jim was able to gain some insight into his negativity and pessimism. He realized that his current reaction to the book letdown was similar to the way he'd reacted to disappointments and insecurities he'd experienced as a child. To avoid the discomfort of any more disappointments, he was seeing everything in the future as negative—that way there would be no surprises.

To help Jim regain his optimism, his therapist suggested he refocus his attention on his "day job." He helped Jim learn ways to rediscover what had excited him about practicing trial law when he started out. Jim also decided to do something fun he had put off for years—he enrolled in a creative art class. He found that painting allowed him to express his creative side without the stress of trying to get a book published. His wife and friends said his paintings were really good. Jim was beginning to think so, too. Hey, maybe one of the local galleries would be interested in showing his early oils . . . In fact, Jim seemed to recall Matisse was a lawyer before he became a famous artist.

A recent study from Wake Forest University found that when we make a conscious effort to experience joy and happiness, it pays off. Dr. Will Fleeson and colleagues found that study volunteers actually felt happier when they *acted* more extroverted—singing aloud, walking over and talking to someone, or being more assertive and energetic—and other people perceived them as happier, too.

Psychotherapists use several approaches to help patients minimize negative thinking. In *cognitive therapy*, negativity is seen as resulting from conscious, negative assumptions and thoughts. Patients are taught to recognize their habitual negative thoughts and learn ways to break the habit.

By learning new cognitive skills, pessimists can, in fact, become more optimistic. Drs. Martin Seligman, Albert Ellis, and others have described systematic cognitive approaches for learning optimism. Generally, a person first focuses on how a particular event triggers a negative feeling in them. They learn to recognize the assumptions they make about those feelings, and the consequences and outcomes of their responses to those feelings. For example, your boss chooses another executive to handle a new account. You immediately feel hurt and rejected, and assume you are about to be fired. With that unsubstantiated and negative assumption tainting your mood and attitude, your performance at work slides. Your boss eventually calls you into her office tomorrow for "the talk." You spend a sleepless night worrying that you'll be fired at tomorrow's meeting with the boss, when actually she plans to hand another new account to you—possibly one you will value even more.

It's not just events that evoke feelings inside us, but the assumptions we assign to those events: I feel so bad for picking my date up late again—*and* I know she'll never go out with me again because of it. To break negative patterns and outcomes, we need to challenge those assumptions and especially to avoid the tendency to generalize negative thoughts. One error at work doesn't mean your job is in jeopardy; a single traffic citation doesn't lead to losing your driving license; and a minor argument with your spouse doesn't spell divorce. If you tend to think in this generally negative manner, remind yourself of your years of work accomplishments, outstanding driving record, or bonds of love and trust; this may help put such negative thinking into perspective.

It is possible to put concerns, worries, and fears into perspective *before* they get us into a rut of negativity. The following exercise can be helpful.

When doing this exercise, focus on only one feeling or situation at a time, then repeat the exercise for other concerns you may have. Afterward, talking with a friend, spouse, or other empathic listener about the process will often provide even more insight.

Exercise for Staying Positive

1. Think of a situation that brings up anxiety or fear for you. Start out with a simple, daily concern—having a disagreement with a friend, fear of misplacing something, or perhaps being late for work. In your mind, play out the likely outcome of this situation, such as hurt feelings, anger, guilt, sadness, etc.

2. While thinking about this situation and its potential outcome, concentrate on your breathing. Breathe deeply and slowly. As you focus on your rhythmic breathing, feel yourself relaxing—physically and mentally.

3. Continue breathing as you consider the feared situation and try to see the bigger picture: With all the good times you and your friend have spent together, it is unlikely that one spat will unravel that. You will probably find or be able to replace the item you lost. Stepping back, learning to relax, and putting worries into perspective allows you to recover a positive attitude more quickly.

Forgive and Forget

The ability to let go of angry feelings and turn the other cheek lowers stress levels and fosters a positive attitude. Dr. Neal Krause of the University of Michigan found that people who are readily able to forgive others experience enhanced psychological well-being and less depression than grudge-holders. The next time someone wrongs you and triggers feelings of anger, try writing them a candid letter; but after you finish it, put the letter away until the next morning. Often the simple process of writing about feelings helps dissipate them. Reading the letter after a night's sleep frequently provides another dose of perspective that helps distance us from the negative feelings—possibly enough to make sending the letter unnecessary.

Many times we hold on to angry feelings over a confrontation we had with someone long after we forget the details of what the dispute was about. This is common between spouses, long-term friends, partners, and family members. The next time you have trouble forgiving someone, even though you'd like to, keep in mind that over time you probably won't recall the actual quarrel anyway. That realization often helps people to get over their anger. Also, trying to understand what the other person is feeling—guilt, embarrassment, frustration, etc.—may help you empathize with the person's point of view and forgive him or her more readily (see Essential 3).

Sometimes we also need to forgive ourselves. Dwelling on feelings of remorse or guilt for past errors rarely solves problems, and it certainly doesn't make us feel any better. Learning to forgive ourselves and let go of our mistakes allows us to gain wisdom from them and move forward.

Keeping a Positive Spin for Quality Longevity

* Make a conscious effort to be extroverted and energetic—happiness is contagious.
* Forgive yourself and others who wrong you—letting go of grudges lowers stress levels and fosters a positive outlook.
* Build self-esteem by making moral choices. Keep in mind your accomplishments and successes to help rebut your inner self-critic.
* If you don't already have an active spiritual or religious life, consider getting one, whether it's through meditation, organized religion, seeking harmony with nature, or any other form.
* Learn to be optimistic through simple, systematic approaches. Recognize what your negativity triggers are, and challenge any negative assumptions you are quick to make.
* Avoid pessimistic thinking by focusing on your strengths and setting achievable and realistic goals.
* Don't be a loner—ask others for support and get professional help if you need it.

Essential 3

Cultivate Healthy and Intimate Relationships

Friendship is born at that moment when one person says to another, "What! You too? I thought I was the only one."

—C. S. LEWIS

Shirley I. was finally taking her long-awaited getaway from her patients, daughter, boyfriend, parents, and friends. She had an experienced psychologist covering for her, and her daughter knew how to reach her in case of an emergency. This was *her* week to chill out at her favorite spa—catch up on her reading and not answer to anyone about anything. She warned them all that morning: "If it's not life or death, don't call me—I don't want to talk to *anybody* for seven days!" Once she got to the spa, Shirley stashed her cell phone, turned off her BlackBerry, and hid behind her giant sunglasses as she settled in at the pool with a novel.

"Hi, mind if we take this lounger?" Shirley glanced up at two smiling young women. "Sure, go ahead," Shirley said, and then went back to reading as the ladies spread their towels on the lounge chairs next to hers and chatted as they ordered drinks from a passing waiter, put suntan lotion on each other's backs, and got out their own books to read. Shirley noticed the blond woman's book and said, "I read that one. I loved it." The blonde smiled. "Really? Thank goodness. I hate going on a trip without a really good book." Shirley sat up. "Me, too. I mean, I've been so excited about getting away for a week of solitude, I actually brought six books just in case I didn't like any of them." All three women laughed. "That's why I love this place! I can really relax here and be alone. I am so exhausted from dealing with everyone in my life that my jaws actually hurt from talking. I'm Shirley, by the way." They introduced themselves all around and continued to chitchat. When the drinks came, Shirley put them on her tab and ordered everybody lunch as they continued to gab.

Humans are naturally social. We not only enjoy being with others, we thrive on it. Our need for intimacy, emotional connectedness, and social support begins in infancy and lasts for the rest of our lives. Dr. Rene Spitz and others found that a high proportion of adequately nourished infants who were not held or caressed by their mothers frequently experienced developmental delays.

Adults have a similar need for contact. Research has shown that people exposed to periods of sensory deprivation, such as prisoners in solitary confinement, may hallucinate and lose their ability to differentiate between fantasy and reality. It is critical to our well-being that we remain intimately connected—through talking, touching, and relating honestly to people we care about. Anyone experiencing quality longevity will credit healthy and intimate relationships as among the most meaningful and important elements of their life.

Social Butterflies Live Longer

Dr. Thomas Glass and his associates at Harvard University showed that spending enjoyable time with others actually extends life expectancy. They looked at approximately three thousand older

Americans to see how much time they spent in a variety of social activities, such as playing games, attending sports events, and going out to restaurants. Their decade of research showed that the chance of longer survival was 20 percent *greater* for people who spent more time socializing than for those who socialized very little or not at all.

Several recent studies have demonstrated the direct *physical* benefits of social support. Dr. Elizabeth Brondolo and her colleagues at St. John's University in New York City studied a group of the city's traffic officers as they faced the daily stress of confronting violators and issuing tickets. They looked at how the repeated threats and insults from disgruntled drivers affected the officers' blood pressure and other physical measures, and whether or not receiving support and encouragement from their colleagues would reduce these stress effects.

By monitoring the officers' physical responses throughout the day, the researchers found that job stress spiked blood pressure. However, when colleagues offered friendly support, especially during high-tension moments, blood pressure remained stable.

Staying connected reduces anxiety and lowers the amount of stress hormones released into the body. This is important because stress hormones are known to contribute to heart disease, diabetes, Alzheimer's, and many other age-related diseases. The MacArthur Study of Successful Aging found that long-standing emotional support was associated with significantly lower blood levels of cortisol and other stress hormones. Socially connected volunteers in that study also required less pain medication following surgery, recovered more quickly, and followed their doctor's post-op advice more closely.

When we are close to a group of people, it makes us feel part of something and gives us a sense of belonging. It lifts our spirits and builds self-esteem. There are practical benefits as well—friends, family members, coworkers, and neighbors are there for each other, available to help each other out if needed. Whether it's borrowing a cup of detergent or getting a ride to the auto mechanic, it's nice to have others to lean on.

Good Habits Are Catchy

We usually meet and get to know people through a common denominator—we are parents at the same school, neighbors on the same block, or coworkers at the same company—so we're predisposed to having at least one or more things in common. Just how much influence any individual or group has upon us depends on our prior experiences with them, as well as our history of relationships with others. Social scientists describe an "inner circle"—the people whom we consider closest to us, usually spouses, children, siblings, or other close family and friends. For most of us, the size of this influential inner circle, whether it includes a spouse or several friends and relatives, tends to remain stable over the years, even if the people in that circle change.

When we spend a significant amount of time with certain people, we tend to adopt and share the same attitudes and lifestyle habits. Often we don't realize the impact these lifestyle influences are making on the quality of our longevity. If we surround ourselves with a health-conscious crowd, we are perhaps more likely to meet for a game of golf on a Sunday morning rather than a Saturday afternoon of cocktails and munchies at the club lounge.

Kimberly L., a forty-two-year-old personal stylist, met Richard T., an architect, at her tennis club. He was charming and funny, and she hadn't met anyone else she wanted to date in almost a year. At first he joined her in tennis and hiking, her favorite pastimes, but that soon gave way to late-night dinners and parties with Richard's large circle of friends.

Kimberly enjoyed being with Richard, but the more time she spent with him, the less time she spent at the tennis court, hiking trail, or gym. She began losing sleep and gaining a few pounds, and she'd even been late for work a couple of times. Her best friend, Alice, mentioned that she was looking a bit worse for wear.

One evening as they finished a late supper at a French restaurant, Richard suggested that they go to his favorite bar for a nightcap. Kimberly said she'd had enough to drink for a weeknight and perhaps they should go home and try to make it to the gym in the morning. Richard got defensive and said he didn't need a "mommy" to tell him what to do. Not wanting to start an argument, Kimberly gave in and joined Richard for a drink with his friends.

The next morning Kimberly woke up a little hungover and was late for work. After a long talk with Alice, Kimberly decided to give Richard an ultimatum: Either they lighten up on the partying, or they stop seeing each other. Richard got angry and said, "Fine. Let's take a break." Kimberly was hurt, but she stuck to her guns. The first few days were rough, but she knew she was doing the best thing for herself, and Alice was there to lend support.

A week later, Richard called and apologized. He said he missed her and was ready to clean up his act. He asked if they could meet sometime for a round of tennis. Kimberly said sure, and she'd buy the drinks afterward—at the smoothie bar.

As in Kimberly's case, we can often influence others just as they can influence us. Some of us have advised our children to choose their friends wisely, and perhaps we could benefit from that same wisdom.

Clearing Out Relationship Clutter

Sometimes we hold on to relationships long after they become not just nonessential, but detrimental or even toxic. Unhealthy relationships can complicate our lives and lead us to repeat negative patterns that can bring on frustration and guilt. When we have too many of these toxic friendships or even one that has become prominent in our lives, we suffer from *relationship clutter*. It may be time to clean house—emotionally.

Clearing out relationship clutter often requires spending less time with some individuals and more with others, or perhaps severing an unhealthy relationship completely. If an acquaintance places unreasonable and heavy demands on our time and resources, it can consume our energy and leave us emotionally drained.

Sometimes people remain in unhealthy relationships simply out of habit. The negativity or uncomfortable feelings from the toxic friendship may have been going on for so long that they don't even realize they *can* unburden themselves from the feelings by getting distance from the other person. Once we change or sever such a relationship, the reduction in stress alone can go a long way toward improving the quality of our longevity.

On the other hand, it is possible to reenergize a relationship with someone when it has gotten off track. The surest way to reconnect with someone is by carving out some dedicated time to be together—alone—during which both people can share their thoughts and feelings. When deciding whether or not to try to repair a friendship, you might consider how long you've known the person, if you

Barbara and Greg W., midfifties, were coming up on their thirtieth anniversary. While they were out to dinner with old friends Jane and Alan, Jane insisted on helping them plan a big party to celebrate their anniversary—especially since Barbara and Greg had done "absolutely nothing" to mark their twenty-fifth. Clearly, Jane didn't consider Barbara and Greg's romantic twenty-fifth-anniversary trip to Rome as very significant. Jane said the party *had* to be at the new luxurious hotel she had just decorated—the caterer was to die for! And they *had* to start working on the guest list ASAP!

That night Barbara was all fired up about Jane's party idea: She'd have to get a new outfit, and Greg would definitely need a new suit. Oh, and did she mention that Jane knew the most fabulous stationer to make the invitations? Greg put up his hands. "Whoa, there. Weren't we going to spend our anniversary visiting the kids? I thought you wanted to play with your new granddaughter?" "I *do!*" Barbara said defensively. "We'll just fly all the kids out here for a week. That's what Jane and Alan did. It'll be great!" Greg glanced around the sleek and modern condo they had downsized to after their youngest was out of the house and married, and wasn't so sure. And, except for their daughters' weddings, he and Barbara had never been so keen on throwing big parties.

Over the next two weeks, Jane put Barbara through an abridged version of "Party Planning 101"—menus, flowers, music, invitations, and the most important thing of all: compiling the guest list. Barbara either couldn't make up her mind or didn't really care about many of the details, so she left several decisions in the willing hands of Jane. The bills, however, were placed wholly and firmly onto Barbara's credit cards, and Greg was *not happy* with the situation.

One night, as Barbara was getting ready for bed, Greg lay propped up, reviewing the bills. "You booked a photographer for fifteen hundred dollars? Why can't your sister take the pictures? She's good with a camera." Barbara replied from the bathroom, "This guy shot Jane's son's wedding! He's incredible! We're lucky to get him!" Greg mumbled something about his "great luck" as Barbara got into bed and said, "I just hope we can fit everyone into the Terrace Ballroom at the hotel." Greg took a deep breath. "Just how many people are we talking about?" Barbara took out the guest list Jane had printed out for her. "Hopefully no more than 150." Greg reached for the list. "May I see that?" He looked it over. "You're inviting the Franks? We haven't even spoken to them in maybe three years." Barbara got defensive. "Judy Frank goes to the same hairdresser as Jane, so she's going to know about the party. And I have to invite Jane's sister and brother-in-law, and her parents, too. They can sit with Dr. Robertson." Greg was dumbfounded. "Our old pediatrician?!" Pouting, Barbara responded, "He was Jane's pediatrician, too! And they're still really close!"

Greg continued to peruse the list, annoyed. "I thought you didn't like Christine Fowler. Didn't you say she was a mean-spirited gossip queen?" Barbara snorted. "She is. But I'd rather have her out broadcasting what a great party I had instead of what a witch I was for not inviting her." Greg sighed. "That sounds like Jane talking." Barbara turned away, angry, turned off her bedside lamp, and started to cry. Greg put down the list and took her in his arms. "I'm sorry, honey. I know you've been working really hard on this thing, and I didn't mean to upset you." She sniffed. "I know. It's okay. I guess I'm just stressed out. Putting this thing together, spending all this money, having all the kids and the grandkids coming here—I just feel overwhelmed." Greg kissed her lightly. "It's *our* thirtieth anniversary, honey. We can always blow off this shindig and run away to some tropical paradise . . ." Barbara turned to face him. "Are you kidding? Jane would never speak to me again!"

The following week was another whirlwind of activity surrounding the party—airline flights had to be booked for the kids, clothes had to be tailored, shopping had to be done, and home repairs had to be completed. On Friday afternoon, Jane called Barbara and announced that she needed to add four more people to the guest list—the Kleins and the Ruperts from the tennis club—they all just adored Barbara and Greg, and Jane just *had* to invite them to the party. Barbara balked. "Jane, the maximum for the Terrace Room is 160, and we're already at that." Jane took a moment, then calmly said, "Barbara, darling, your sister and her family haven't committed yet. That's six people! And they live three thousand miles away, for Pete's sake. You don't *have* to encourage them to come . . ." Barbara was shocked. "But she's my *sister*. She was maid of honor at my wedding. I *want* her there." Jane, unfazed, replied, "Just offering a suggestion, doll. Take it or leave it."

That night, Barbara decided to leave it. The next day she and Greg called the stationers, the florist, the hotel, and the photographer, and were able to retrieve most of their deposit money. Barbara's stress melted away as she came to realize that the party had become more about Jane's need to be a social butterfly, and less about Barbara and Greg celebrating their thirty years of love and commitment. They didn't need the Kleins or the Ruperts, or a demanding pushy friend to remind them of what was important and worth honoring in their lives.

Two days before their anniversary, Barbara and Greg boarded a plane for the East Coast to visit their kids and grandchildren. Barbara's sister's family—all six of them—drove down for a night of celebration. Then the whole clan saw Barbara and Greg off on their romantic tropical voyage to the Bahamas. Barbara remembered to bring her "A" list of people to send island postcards to, and neither the Kleins nor the Ruperts made the cut.

and this person have been successful at resolving differences in the past, and whether or not this person has been or will be a positive influence in your life.

Any real and satisfying relationship takes time to nurture, and for most of us, time is limited. We need to make wise choices about the people we spend our precious free time with—and, ideally, choose people with whom we can have mutually nurturing relationships.

Empathy: The Basic Social Skill

To imaginatively see things from another person's perspective and be able to understand his or her feelings is commonly known as "empathy." The ability to convey this understanding back to the other person is the emotional glue that keeps us socially connected. With empathy, we feel less alone in the world and are able to build closeness, friendship, and love.

By participating in groups that empathize together, and share a common cause, goal, or purpose, we become part of a social network. College fraternities, book clubs, alumni associations, school PTAs, charity boards, neighborhood watch committees, and political action groups are just a few examples of the ways in which people group together around similar empathic interests.

Social networks can increase our sense of belonging, purpose, and self-worth, all of which promote a positive outlook. They can help us get through difficult and stressful times, such as a divorce, a job loss, or the death of a loved one, as well as the happy types of stressful times, such as a wedding or the birth of a baby. And we don't necessarily have to lean on family and friends for support to reap the benefits. Simply knowing they're available can give us a sense of confidence when we face stressful events or other problems.

Scientists recently found that helping other people actually improves the helper's mental and physical health. Study volunteers who mentored young children experienced greater physical strength and stamina, better social interaction, and more mental stimulation than a control group that was not mentoring.

Some people are natural-born empathizers. They instantly put their own needs aside in order to be emotionally available for a friend or family member. However, not everyone is heavily weighted with this gift. Many of us have to make more of an effort, especially when distracted by the seemingly never-ending complications of our own lives. Although we'd like to think we would drop everything for a friend in need, it might require some effort to give up floor seats to a basketball playoff game the moment your friend calls and wants to spend a few hours talking about being stood up for a date.

Most of us know one or more people who seem to have no empathy skills at all, and were it not for work, family, or social obligations, we might choose to avoid these people altogether. This kind of person typically does not listen nor remember what we've told them, or even what they've told us. They appear unmoved by other people's suffering and unable or unwilling to share in their joy. It is hard to feel connected to those who lack in empathy, and they are often labeled as bores or narcissists. Luckily, most people — even the empathy-challenged — can improve their skills with a little work and some simple techniques.

We first begin learning empathy as infants by observing it in our parents. They nurture and care for us, which helps us develop our sense of self and ability to identify with and relate to others. From our parents' caring caresses, understanding words, smiles, nods, and other nonverbal communications, we learn to regulate our own emotional responses. These early experiences help shape our ability to get close to others on an emotional level.

As we mature and become more independent, we turn away

from our parents and look to get our "empathy fix" from like-minded peers who share our interests, desires, and values. Eventually, we develop more intimate relationships outside of the family and aspire to deeper levels of sustained empathy in marriage and other long-term relationships.

The powerful form of loving empathy that jolts many of us when we have our own children leads us to an intense closeness and bonding with our kids. Most parents would sacrifice their own lives instantly to protect their children.

Many people agree that one of the most effective ways we become empathic toward others is by experiencing our own pain, loss, or elation. Anyone who has lived through the death of a sibling, spouse, or parent knows all too well how difficult it is for someone else going through that same experience. On the other hand, knowing the joy of holding your first child or grandchild, or perhaps watching your eldest daughter get married, is a feeling that is wonderful to share with a friend who may be experiencing it for the first time.

Our capacity for empathy is often challenged when our parents age and we are thrust into the unfamiliar role of caring for them. Although it can be emotionally confusing to care for the people who have always cared for us, many adult children lovingly care for their parents if the need arises.

Empathy has likely given the human species an edge in natural selection. Our ancient ancestors' empathy gave them connective social glue that provided a survival advantage against the adversities of their environment. By banding together, they were better able to fend off predators and nurture their offspring, whereas alone they would have been less likely to survive. Current science indicates that our social connectedness has more than a survival advantage — it has a biological basis as well.

Hardwired to Connect

With recent neuroimaging studies, doctors are discovering what appears to be the hardwiring of empathy in our brains. Dr. Tania Singer and her team studied couples in love at the Institute of Neurology at University College in London. They measured brain activity in volunteer couples when one partner experienced a pain stimulus, such as a brief electric shock. That person later observed their partner appear to be experiencing the same brief pain. Whether a volunteer actually felt the painful stimulus or whether they believed their lover felt it didn't matter. The same emotional brain centers were triggered, suggesting that these emotional brain centers may be the root of empathic experiences.

We don't have to be in love to experience empathy. Just seeing someone's facial expression—whether it's painful or pleasurable— sets off a sophisticated network of neuronal wires that fires the message through a preset pathway and triggers a response in us. This brain hardwiring for emotion is not set in stone, and we can exert some control over what we feel. Neuroscientists at the UCLA Ahmanson Lovelace Brain Mapping Center found that when volunteers observed emotional facial expressions, certain brain areas lit up on their MRI scans. Afterward, by simply imitating those emotional facial expressions, the volunteers were able to light up the identical brain areas on their MRIs.

These findings are in line with the earliest concepts of empathy. When the German psychologist Theodore Lipps originally coined the term in the late nineteenth century, he postulated that we actually imitate another person's actions when we empathize. This "chameleon effect" has been observed in empathic individuals when they unconsciously mimic mannerisms and facial expressions of others, as opposed to people who show little empathy—sometimes referred to as "stone-faced."

Higher Education in Empathy

In school, we are taught a variety of subjects, from reading and writing to physical education and even music appreciation. But as yet, there is no standard curriculum on empathy to help us communicate effectively with important people in our lives.

Empathy, however, is becoming widely accepted as an ability that can be learned in order to enhance our social connectedness. It strengthens our sense of closeness and fulfillment in our relationships. We begin learning empathy, like language, during early childhood. And just like language, we can continue to hone those skills throughout our lifetime. The empathy process involves several components that can be fine-tuned with practice.

RECOGNIZING OTHER PEOPLE'S FEELINGS

By age twelve, most of us are aware of our own various emotions and can recognize those same emotions in others. We can learn to empathize with others by drawing upon our own experiences that were similar to what the other person appears to be going through.

Some people have more trouble differentiating among subtle emotional states. The ability to recognize the subtleties of facial expression as well as body and verbal language can be learned, practiced, and improved upon. Some psychologists have their patients view and study photographs or drawings that convey a range of facial expressions of various emotions such as anger, guilt, fear, or sadness, to help them learn to recognize those emotions. Once we are able to recognize another person's emotional state, we can more readily empathize with that person's feelings.

ATTENTIVE LISTENING

When we are engaged in a conversation, it's natural to want to jump in when a thought or reaction gets triggered in us. However, interrupting somebody in midsentence or midthought may distract or frustrate that person, and we could end up not hearing how they really feel. Great conversationalists are often people who say little, but listen a great deal. Empathic individuals tend to give the other person enough time to relate their experience as fully as possible. This type of attentive listening requires self-control—not just over interrupting the speaker or allowing your mind to wander, but also over unnecessary movement or fidgeting that can distract the speaker.

The following exercise not only helps build listening skills, it can be used as a regular tool to "check in" with your partner or close friend after a long day or other period of time apart. Sometimes just five minutes of uninterrupted attentive listening is all it takes to connect with someone you have been merely passing rushing in the hallway for days—even if you live under the same roof.

Attentive Listening Exercise

This exercise can help us learn to avoid being distracted by our own thoughts and reactions, including the desire to jump in and participate while the other person is speaking. You can do this exercise with a friend, spouse, family member, or even someone you don't know very well. Set aside fifteen minutes so you both can take a turn.

- *One Person Talks.* **For three to five minutes, one partner talks about something that is going on in his or her life right now. It could be a crisis,** chronic issue, or perhaps a past or upcoming event. Beginners may choose to start by discussing feelings or situations that do not involve the listener directly. If the topic does involve the listener, the speaker should be careful to discuss only his or her *feelings* about the situation, individual, or relationship, and avoid criticizing the listener. This exercise is *not* about attacking and defending, it is about talking, listening, and being understood.

- *Other Person Listens.* The listener should not interrupt or coax. Rather than jump in and say, "I know just what you mean! I've felt exactly like that!" the listener should maintain eye contact and stay focused on what the other person is saying. Even if the listener's mind wanders momentarily to thoughts like, "What am I going to say when it's my turn?" the listener should push those thoughts away and bring his or her attention back to what the speaker is saying.

- *Switch Roles.* After three to five minutes, the *listener* now talks about something he or she is going through, and the other person becomes the attentive listener. The topic may be completely unrelated to the first speaker's discussion. If it is related to the first person's discussion, the second speaker should be careful not to retaliate or attack, and instead focus on his or her own feelings.

- *Discuss the Experience.* After both partners have had a chance to speak and listen, they should spend the next few minutes discussing what the experience felt like. Many people find that by simply listening attentively, they develop an al-

> most immediate sense of empathy and under-
> standing for the other person. By being listened
> to thoughtfully, most people feel understood and
> cared about. It may take practice to break the
> habit of interrupting the speaker with encourag-
> ing thoughts, feelings, and one's own experi-
> ences, but it gets easier with practice.

COMMUNICATING YOUR EMPATHIC RESPONSE

Understanding what another person is going through is a large part of empathy. *Conveying* that understanding back to the other person is just as important, and is what truly draws people together and keeps them close. Communicating with another person about his or her concerns, without criticizing, makes that person feel understood. This kind of exchange involves basic communication skills—both verbal and nonverbal—including eye contact, facial expression, and body language. Even people who are born great communicators can enhance these skills.

One way to communicate your understanding after attentively listening is to clarify what you heard the other person tell you. You could try saying things like, "I want to make sure I understand this . . ." or "Let's see if I have this right." You can then restate the other person's feelings or situation and try to paraphrase their words. Asking for more detail is also helpful. Follow-up questions show the other person that you have heard them, you're interested, and you would like to know more.

If your partner is trying to cope with a difficult situation, you might start by acknowledging his or her efforts. If there is nothing you can do to help, let your partner know that you understand and are willing to listen. Sometimes just lending a nonjudgmental ear can be far more supportive than trying to fix the situation.

Communicating our understanding and compassion to our mates not only brings us closer, but can also enhance our sexual fulfillment. A satisfying sex life contributes to overall quality longevity—physically and emotionally—and really brings people together.

Good Sex for Longer Life

Researchers the world over have reported a positive link between sexual activity and life expectancy. A recent study determined the level of sexual activity of nearly one thousand men from a town in South Wales, and then followed their health outcomes over the next ten years. The life expectancy for the sexually active men—those reporting orgasms twice or more each week—was 50 percent greater than for the men who experienced orgasms less than once a month.

One of the longevity-increasing benefits of remaining sexually active may be its association with lower rates of heart attacks, which researchers speculate is related to the release of the hormone DHEA during orgasm. Testosterone, the hormone that stimulates sex drive in both women and men, has been found to help reduce the risk of heart attack, as well. Sexual activity also helps maintain physical fitness by burning calories and fat.

Engaging in sexual activity may also bolster immune function, the body's ability to fight off infection. A study of college students found 30 percent higher immunoglobulin A levels in those having sexual intercourse once or twice a week, as compared with abstinent students. (Of course, this doesn't apply to my own teenage daughter, who will have no time for such activities due to constant studying and then conducting the New York Philharmonic Orchestra, until she marries the perfect young man who meets my complete approval.)

Research shows that besides improving physical health and potentially adding years to one's life, healthy sexual activity adds quality to those years, as well. Sexual satisfaction reduces tension and helps us sleep better, perhaps through the release of endorphins and other hormones. Studies have also found it to relieve chronic back pain, anxiety, and headaches. Positive sexual experiences often increase self-esteem, and many religions and cultures view sexual expression as a tool for spiritual enlightenment.

Love the One You're With

A healthy sex life fosters intimacy, feelings of affection, and closeness between partners. Expressing our sexual desire is a basic ingredient in bonding as a couple, and sexually satisfied couples have a greater probability of long-term stability.

Although sexual intimacy is good for our health, emotional state, and longevity forecast, many people find it challenging to keep passion alive over the course of several years. Family needs, work pressures, illnesses, and a multitude of distractions may leave some people physically exhausted and emotionally depleted at the end of the day, and sex may be the last thing on their minds. The following simple strategies can help couples communicate better, strengthen intimacy, and ultimately lead to a more satisfying sex life.

FIRST, LOVE THE ONE YOU ARE

It's very easy to blame a partner for his or her lack of sexual interest. Because he or she no longer dresses or acts sexy, initiates intimate contact, or perhaps even mentions sex, our own desire has shut down.

Before pointing at a partner, however, one should try focusing on oneself. Letting go of negative feelings like anger, guilt, and fear gives us a more positive outlook and helps bolster our sexual self-esteem. As we age, our bodies change, but it is a myth that sexual quality and desire necessarily decline. In fact, as we gain more experience and wisdom, lovemaking can become more pleasurable than ever before. By practicing mindful awareness—staying in the moment and remaining aware of all the sensations going on in our bodies—we are likely to be more playful and emotionally available to our partner, which in turn can help our partner to overcome his or her own distractions and fears.

TALKING SEX

Talking with a partner about sexual desires and fantasies can be difficult, especially when one is unaccustomed to doing so. But the benefits can be so great that a little discomfort is usually well worth the effort. Partners might start by discussing sexual experiences they have had together that were particularly satisfying. Try the following simple exercise:

1. Tell your partner something he or she has done in the past that really turned you on. Your partner may not be aware that it was so enjoyable for you.
2. Your partner now tells you something you have done that really turned him or her on.

This kind of discussion can begin a sexual dialogue that leads to sharing of fantasies and more fulfilling sexual intimacy.

SHOW THAT YOU LISTENED

Responding positively and nonjudgmentally to your partner's sexual wishes promotes greater intimacy. If you have told your partner about something that excites you in bed and he or she responds by trying it, you know that your partner has listened, cares, and wants to please you. That's as good a description of love as any. Whether it's lighting a few candles, buying new sexy pajamas, or massaging your partner's back, taking the initiative is another way to show your partner that you are interested and want to please him or her.

MORE TIPS ON STAYING INTIMATELY CONNECTED

Even the closest of couples may find that the challenges of work and family can leave them mentally and physically exhausted by day's end—thus derailing their goal of being sexually intimate with each other. There are several positive steps people can take to overcome these and other common barriers that sometimes arise in relationships. Consider some of these suggestions:

Schedule an intimate date. Plan ahead for time alone with your partner—perhaps dinner at your favorite restaurant followed by a romantic night at a hotel, or even a cozy evening at home alone. The anticipation alone can be exciting.

Set the mood. Before going to bed, spruce up the bedroom with some candles, play soft music, and if you enjoy incense, light some.

Time your medicines. Many of us experience aches and pains that may restrict our movement and distract us from "the mood." Discover the time it takes for your medicine to take effect—whether it's an anti-inflammatory, a sexual-function enhancer, or even a Tylenol—and be sure to take it accordingly.

Try a "quickie." Not all lovemaking has to be a major event preceded by candlelit dinners and roses. Sometimes a brief sexual encounter—complete with excitement and urgency—can be a spicy variation. Whether it is a spontaneous encounter in the bathroom while the kids are watching TV, or a brief midday rendezvous at lunch, these get-togethers often have a fun and sneaky quality that can be exhilarating.

Indulge your fantasies. Try telling your partner some private thoughts that turn you on. Almost everyone has sexual fantasies and exploring them with your partner can bring you to a new level of intimacy.

The Value of Vows

According to information from the Centers for Disease Control and Prevention, marriage may increase life expectancy by as much as five years. Numerous studies have found that married people live longer, happily married people live the longest, and married couples who continue to be sexually active (with each other, of course) are *most* satisfied with their lives, overall.

New research from the University of Warwick in England found that a spouse's happiness spills over to the partner's state of mind. The study looked at over 9,700 married couples and compared them to 3,300 couples who lived together out of wedlock. A happier husband made for a happier wife and vice versa, but this did not hold true for the unmarried couples. The study showed that the cohabitating couples who remained unmarried had a greater sense of personal autonomy at the cost of their emotional connection.

The national divorce rate has nearly doubled during the last forty years, and a growing industry of "marriage educators" has attempted to remedy today's fractured families. Typically, there are three types of couples-counseling techniques that assist partners in improving their communication skills and satisfaction with their relationships. In the traditional and most common technique, behavioral marital therapy, the therapist helps the couple learn communication skills and ways to resolve their differences in a kinder, more empathic manner. A second form, insight-oriented marital therapy, uses both behavioral techniques and strategies for understanding the other person's reasons for becoming angry and defensive in the relationship, in order to defuse chronic power struggles.

A third, newer approach—emotionally focused therapy—helps people recognize that their partner has needs and coping styles that may differ greatly from their own. Partners learn to appreciate and accommodate these differences, rather than attempting to change them. Dr. Susan Johnson of the University of Ottawa has studied this form of relatively brief therapy—usually eight to twelve sessions—and has found significant gains that last at least three years for most couples, even those at high risk for divorce. This is a much higher success rate than that reported for the more traditional forms of couples therapy.

Many couples don't need formal therapy to help resolve their conflicts and keep their relationships on track. However, even contented, successful couples can benefit from some simple strategies to help them stay connected and happy for the long haul.

Set aside time. Many people are so busy multitasking throughout their waking hours that they may have little time left to talk about their day-to-day concerns and personal issues with their partner. Make it a daily ritual to spend some time together—without kids, friends, television, or other distractions. This time can be used to talk about what's on your mind and how you're really feeling. Sometimes just holding your partner and *not* talking may be what is needed.

Keep a sense of humor. All couples argue. What defines a successful marriage is *how* the couple argues. Try to punctuate a disagreement with an occasional smile or some humor to convey your understanding of the other person's idiosyncrasies.

Stay in touch. An effective way to maintain emotional closeness during a period apart can be a quick phone call or voice mail to let your partner know you are thinking about them. An e-mail works well, too.

Don't criticize. Focusing solely on your partner's weaknesses may make him or her defensive and sabotage your attempts to feel connected. Try talking about the feelings that your partner's actions trigger in you, rather than simply criticizing his or her actions. Instead of saying, "Why do you have to be so thoughtless and slam the door while I am working?" try "When you slam the door while I'm working, I lose my train of thought and I feel frustrated and powerless."

Socialize as a couple. Find things you and your partner like going out and doing together, and try to do them with other people you enjoy spending time with—particularly other like-minded couples. Sharing views and new ideas with other people carries over into your own relationship and keeps things lively—even if it's only a few private laughs after everyone else has gone home.

Take care of yourself. Most people in long-term relationships understand that their partner cannot meet all of their personal needs. Besides taking responsibility for your own medical health, you need to care for yourself emotionally and socially. Regular tennis games, poker nights, book clubs, support groups, community theater, sporting leagues, and involvement with religious or charity groups are just a few of the ways we can refuel ourselves independently of our partners. When we come back together, we are often emotionally energized and ready to enjoy each other's company.

Table for One

Most people spend a good portion of their adult lives as single people, whether they're unmarried, divorced, or widowed. And despite progress in defining the individual with greater independence in today's society, there is still an emphasis on couples, as well as security in groups. If you've ever eaten at a table for one at a fine restaurant, you may know how it feels—people smile sympathetically or act like you're contagious, while the waiters constantly inquire, "Will someone else be joining you?"

Coupling is not the social solution to quality longevity for everyone. There are advantages to being single and able to make decisions based on one's own needs and desires, without having to compromise to suit another person's whims. But the need for social connectedness remains, and single people who maintain strong relationships with family, friends, and community groups live longer than those who do not. In fact, single women, who tend to have stronger and longer-lasting relationships with friends and family, outlive their male counterparts by several years. It benefits single people to remain out there and connected, whether it's through sports, work, dating, volunteering, or other social activities.

Man's Best Friend

Many people love pets, but most don't realize that pets may contribute to their owners' longer life expectancy. Studies of patients with heart disease have found that pet owners live longer—often more than a year—than those without a pet. A UCLA study showed that dog owners required less medical care for stress-induced aches and pains than the study subjects with no dogs, and these therapeutic effects are not limited to canines. Having cats, parakeets, turtles—even just watching a tank full of tropical fish—have all been shown to lower stress levels, thus contributing to quality longevity.

Some studies have found that pet owners have reduced blood pressure and cholesterol levels, as well as increased life satisfaction levels. Exactly how pets help us reduce stress is not known; however, we definitely bond with our pets, and they can be good and true companions. There are also practical benefits to pet ownership, such as having a walking companion, an alarm that sounds when visitors approach the door, and, as in the case of my dog, a little friend who happily keeps the kitchen floor clear of any food scraps that might happen to fall.

When considering a pet, think about what is practical for you and your family, your living space and surroundings, and your personal preferences. Even people with strong allergies can usually find a hypoallergenic pet they can tolerate and love.

Parent Care

Thanks to advances in medical technology, adult children and their older parents are both enjoying longer life and better health. Still, the risk for chronic disease increases with age, and some adult children, often still dealing with the needs of their own kids, can find themselves simultaneously thrust into the unfamiliar role of caring for their parents.

Because most people continue to look to their parents for emotional support throughout adulthood, it can be psychologically difficult to have that role reversed. For the parents, the idea of turning to their children for help can sometimes be tinged with humiliation.

On a practical level, many older parents and adult children are not prepared to cope with the medical, financial, legal, and geographical challenges that can emerge when parents need the help of their children. It is important to prepare in advance for this possible transition. Most of us who have had a good relationship with our parents and our children want those caring relationships to continue, even if the roles should reverse. Here are some issues and strategies to consider during the transition period associated with parent care.

Be empathic. Parent care may stir up a variety of feelings, such as anxiety, fear, and guilt. Try to anticipate some of the concerns of the other generation. Among the many issues at hand, the adult child needs to consider their parent's possible discomfort about receiving care from them. The parent may want to take into account the sense of loss his or her adult child is experiencing now that the roles are reversing. Remaining empathic will make it easier to talk about mutual feelings and maintain closeness.

Ask for help. Both parents and adult children are often reluctant to ask for help. Parents don't want to burden their children, and many "sandwich-generation" adult children—busy caring for parents and children simultaneously—don't turn to other family members or caregivers for assistance. Traditionally, an adult daughter takes on the greatest responsibility of care, but if she is overburdened and unwilling to let others help, the entire family suffers.

Money matters. Between parents and children, money can be a symbol of love, power, caring, revenge, or a variety of other motives and feelings. Concentrate on clarifying practical questions such as: What are the actual assets and the real needs of the family members? Getting good legal advice on wills, trusts, and other financial issues well in advance of the inter-family discussions of these matters can help families avoid conflicts in the future.

Housing. If a parent can no longer live alone, questions emerge about how to provide the best living arrangement. Some adult children welcome their parents into their homes, which often works out well, especially if the parent has enough privacy and sense of purpose within the family. For others, an assisted-living arrangement or skilled nursing home may be a more feasible alternative. Many resources are available to help families sort through the many alternatives (see Appendix 3).

Health care. Many adult children get involved with their parent's health care if the parent is unable to make all necessary decisions on his or her own. The key is to respect the parent's privacy, yet understand when it's important to step in and help. Having advance directives in place is a good way to make sure the parent's wishes are being followed.

Keeping Relationships Healthy and Intimate

- Stay connected and involved socially, whether you are single or in a couple. Try to spend time with a healthy crowd, because good habits are contagious.
- Clear out relationship clutter by cutting loose unsatisfying or "toxic" friends and acquaintances.
- Develop and maintain your empathy skills. Listen to others, try to identify with their feelings, and let them know that you understand.
- If you are in an intimate relationship, make efforts to nurture it: Schedule time together, share feelings without criticizing, and stay in touch with friends and other couples. A healthy sex life adds to quality longevity.
- Having a pet may contribute to longer life expectancy. Pets can also be enjoyable, stress-reducing companions.
- Planning ahead for the emotional and practical challenges of parent care can make a possible role-reversal much less stressful for both older parents and their adult children.

Essential 4

Promote Stress-Free Living

Reality is the leading cause of stress among those in touch with it.

— LILY TOMLIN

Alan F., fifty-three, gently awakens Monday morning to his favorite classical music station on the clock radio. He feels rested and calm as he recalls the fantastic weekend he spent with his family at the beach. The weather was outstanding, everyone got along great, and he didn't think about his work as a hotel-chain executive at all. During breakfast, Alan promises himself he will *not* let job pressures get to him this week. He's halfway through his shower when the water turns icy cold. Okay, so sharing the hot water is not a concept his kids have yet grasped. He towels off and tells himself it's no big deal, it's still a beautiful morning. Just then he cuts himself shaving—again. Apparently, his wife still hasn't stopped using his razor to shave her legs. Okay, maybe his wife is right and he has a problem sharing, too. His wife, the *expert* sharer, leans in and reminds Alan that he has to stop by the bank today to sign those papers, okay? As he quickly gets dressed, he has no idea how he'll fit the bank into his hectic afternoon. He's already late as he frantically searches for his keys, which are next to his cell phone—which has a dead battery. The housekeeper must have unplugged the charger again when she vacuumed yesterday. Fine, he tells himself, no problem, he'll just charge it at work. Finally, he's relaxing in traffic to the classical music station, dodging between lanes on the freeway, when he notices the flashing red police lights behind him. Alan mutters a profanity and feels his back muscles tensing up as he pulls over on the shoulder. He hears the radio DJ cheerfully report that the weather at the beach is going to be even better than it was on the weekend. As the policeman walks up to his car, Alan wishes his damn cell phone were charged so he could call in sick and head back to the beach.

Stress—a major contributor to age-related diseases—cannot be avoided entirely. Most people, including Alan F., experience stress from work pressures, annoyances at home, and any number of other daily aggravations. However, by learning to minimize stress, as well as our responses to it, we can begin to limit its impact on our lives and increase our quality longevity.

Stress isn't only due to crises or problems. Sometimes positive events—having a new child in the family, being promoted, or planning a big celebration—can stress us out. Other times it can be a loss—the death of a friend or family member, a physical illness, or perhaps a divorce. Even a trivial incident can set us off, whether it's a passing criticism, a misplaced car key, or a broken fingernail. Whatever the cause, science has shown that stress weakens our bodies and accelerates aging.

Under intense stress, our bodies mobilize energy and release stress hormones such as cortisol. As a result, our heartbeat, blood pressure, and breathing rate increase causing more oxygen to be delivered to our muscles. During this acute reaction, nonessential functions such as digestion are suppressed. This "fight or flight" response is an ideal physiological survival tool and useful in many dangerous situations. However, when stress becomes chronic, constant worry or aggravation can keep this stress response turned on, and the continual release of stress hormones can damage the body.

A recent study found that chronic stress may accelerate the very aging of our cells. Scientists from the University of California in San Francisco found that volunteers with higher stress levels had cellular markers of aging equivalent to at least one decade of additional aging, as compared to low-stress volunteers.

Over time, elevated levels of cortisol and other stress hormones can literally shrink the memory centers in our brains and increase our risk for Alzheimer's disease. Ongoing stress has also been associated with an increased risk for high blood pressure, irregular heartbeats, and some forms of cancer.

A twenty-year study of approximately thirteen thousand people found that chronic stress increased the risk of dying from stroke or heart disease. Stress has been shown to undermine our immune system, which diminishes our ability to fight off colds and infections. For some people, stress affects the digestive system and leads to conditions ranging from ulcers to irritable bowel syndrome. Stress can also raise blood sugar levels—a known risk for developing diabetes. Body weight and obesity rates are increased by chronic stress, because stress can stimulate both the appetite hormone leptin and the mood-altering chemical serotonin.

Although what triggers our stress is often beyond our control, how we perceive a stress-provoking event and the way in which we react to it directly determine its impact on our health. We *can* learn simple stress-reduction techniques to greatly improve our responses to stress and reduce its effects on us. Many of the other essential strategies, such as getting regular exercise and eating well, enjoying healthy relationships, and maintaining a positive outlook, also help reduce stress.

How Stressed Out Are You?

Understanding yourself—what stresses you out the most and how you instinctively react—is a first step to figuring out how to possibly avoid or detoxify your most stressful situations, as well as how to manage your reactions. The symptoms of stress are not always obvious, since they can be both physical and mental. If you can link up the specific stress symptom to the cause of the stress, you have taken a big step toward low-stress living. Answer the following questions to get a better idea of how stressed out you are and what triggers your stress response.

Stress Level Questionnaire

	Low		Medium		High	
How would you rate your overall stress level?	1	2	3 4	5	6	7

To what degree do the following situations make you tense or irritable?

	Little		Somewhat		Very	
Argument with friend or relative	1	2	3 4	5	6	7
Waiting for a table in a restaurant.	1	2	3 4	5	6	7
Arriving late for an appointment	1	2	3 4	5	6	7
Anticipating work deadlines.	1	2	3 4	5	6	7

How easy is it for you to relax when you . . .

	Easy		Medium		Difficult	
Watch a television show or movie	1	2	3 4	5	6	7
Read a book or magazine	1	2	3 4	5	6	7

	Easy	Medium	Difficult

Take a walk, jog, or do other physical
exercise. 1 2 3 4 5 6 7

How often do you experience each of the following?

	Never	Sometimes	Always

Insomnia. 1 2 3 4 5 6 7
Shortness of breath 1 2 3 4 5 6 7
Rapid heart rate. 1 2 3 4 5 6 7
Cold hands or feet. 1 2 3 4 5 6 7
Impatience or irritability. 1 2 3 4 5 6 7
Headaches. 1 2 3 4 5 6 7
Apologizing for snapping at people 1 2 3 4 5 6 7
Tension or worry. 1 2 3 4 5 6 7

Add up your total score, which can range from 16 to 112, and
record it below:

Stress Level Total Score: _____

If your score is less than 40, then your stress levels are manage-
able, but you will still benefit from doing some stress-relief exercises. If you scored between 41 and 80, then you are experiencing
mid-range stress levels. Learning and practicing stress-relieving
techniques will be an essential strategy for improving your quality
longevity. If you scored between 81 and 112, then you are in the
high-stress group and will definitely benefit from the stress-
reduction strategies outlined in this section.

Because people respond differently to the same environmental
stimuli, some individuals seem to cope with stress better than oth-

ers. However, anyone willing to challenge the control stress has on his or her life can lessen its harmful effects. Try the following strategies to lower your stress levels and increase your quality longevity.

Mindful Awareness

Mindful awareness, or mindfulness—the subtle process of moment-to-moment awareness of one's thoughts, feelings, and physical states—is a tool we use to achieve many of the *Longevity Bible* Essentials. By practicing mindful awareness, we are more likely to notice when we have had enough to eat, which helps control body weight. We are able to listen and communicate better, which often improves our relationships. And mindfulness leads to a more positive outlook, which increases our enjoyment of life.

Meditation as a means to achieving mindfulness gained popularity with Westerners when the Beatles and other celebrities began following Maharishi Mahesh Yogi, who founded the Transcendental Meditation movement in the late 1960s. With its roots in ancient Buddhist traditions, mindful awareness is not only the basis of meditation but of many other stress-management techniques as well, including self-hypnosis, biofeedback, and yoga. It also has been used to treat a variety of conditions, including hypertension, chronic pain, and anxiety.

Scientific evidence shows that the act of practiced mindfulness promotes health and mental calm. Systematic EEG brain-wave studies of meditation techniques have found significant effects during and after meditation, as well as improved immune system response to vaccines. And the greater the brain wave changes from meditation, the more effective the immune response. A recent study found that regular meditation increases the size of a brain region that regulates memory and attention. Calming the mind through meditation also appears to improve physical healing. One study found that patients with psoriasis who listened to a meditation tape during ultraviolet light treatments healed four times faster than patients who did not meditate during their treatment.

Meditating on a regular basis may also extend life expectancy. Scientists spent approximately eight years following over two hundred middle-aged and older volunteers with mild forms of high blood pressure—a common illness often worsened by everyday stress. They found that those who meditated regularly had a 23 percent lower mortality rate. Deaths from cardiovascular disease were 30 percent lower and mortality rates from cancer were 49 percent lower in those who meditated, as compared with nonmeditators

Meditation and other forms of mindfulness bring about what Dr. Herbert Benson of Harvard University has termed the relaxation response—a state of deep mental and physical relaxation. Not only does it create a feeling of calm, it alters our physiology: Heart and breathing rates decrease, blood pressure lowers, and muscles relax. Many of these techniques focus on a mantra or a repeated sound that works like a hypnotic rhythm. People are also taught to observe and let go of their habitual mental chatter, and not to focus on distracting body sensations.

The goal is to keep the mind focused on one peaceful thought from moment to moment (see box). It can be frustrating at first, since our minds naturally swing from past ruminations to future worries. Initially, many people get impatient, feeling that they can't stay focused—their minds drift off to mundane thoughts, such as cleaning the garage or what they need from the market. But you needn't reach nirvana each time to benefit from simple mindful awareness exercises. The objective is simply to train yourself to take a rest from your usual ruminations so you can break some of your old, possibly negative or nonproductive thought patterns. When practiced on a daily basis, it will likely improve your state of mind, general health, and life expectancy.

Meditation Break

To jump-start your path into this ancient practice, pick a mantra—a sound, word, or phrase that is comforting to you, whether it is "world peace," "love," "hmm," "om," or whatever soothes you. Sit in a chair or cross-legged on the floor and rest your hands on your upper thighs, palms up. Close your eyes, relax your muscles, and breathe slowly and naturally. With each exhale, repeat your mantra silently to yourself. Try to keep focused on your mantra and your breathing, and ignore the impulse to let your mind wander. If outside thoughts do drift into your mind— "Did I mail that letter?" "Did I return that phone call?"—don't fret over it; allow those thoughts to drift through and away as you return to your mantra. The more you practice, the easier it will become to allow outside thoughts to pass through quickly. After about five minutes, open your eyes and sit quietly for another minute or so, as you ease yourself back into your day. Do this exercise daily and build up to ten-minute sessions.

Multitasking—Minds Under Stress

The term "multitasking" originally referred to a computer's ability to carry out several tasks simultaneously. For many people, multitasking has become a way of life and even a key to success. In fact, some excellent mental aerobic exercises involve engaging the brain in two or more challenging activities at a time. Although checking one's portable e-mail device while talking on a cell phone and reading the newspaper may be second nature for some people (not advisable while driving), many times multitasking can make us less productive, rather than more. And studies show that too much multitasking can lead to increased stress, anxiety, attention deficits, and memory loss.

In order to multitask, the brain uses an area known as the pre-frontal cortex. This "executive" brain center controls our ability to assess and prioritize various tasks. Ironically, chronic stress causes its greatest damage to this prefrontal cortex. Brain scans of volunteers performing multiple tasks together show that as they shift from task to task, this front part of the brain actually takes a moment of rest between tasks. You may have experienced a prefrontal cortex "moment of rest" yourself if you've ever dialed a phone number and suddenly forgotten who you called when the line is answered. What probably occurred is that between the dialing and the answering, your mind shifted to another thought or task, and then took that "moment" to come back. Research has also shown that for many volunteers, job efficiency declines while multitasking, as compared to when they perform only one task at a time.

Multitasking is easiest when at least one of the tasks is routine, habitual, or requires little thought. Most people don't find it difficult to eat and read the newspaper at the same time. However, when two or more attention-requiring tasks are attempted simultaneously, people sometimes get sloppy or make mistakes.

We often don't remember things as well when we're trying to manage several details simultaneously. Without mental focus, we may not pay enough attention to new information coming in, so it never makes it into our memory stores (see Essential 1). That is one of the main reasons we forget people's names—even sometimes right after they have introduced themselves. Multitasking can also affect our relationships. If someone checks their e-mail while on the phone with a friend, they may come off as distracted or disinterested. It can also cause that person to miss or overlook key information being relayed to them.

For chronic multitaskers, I suggest that you schedule a regular time or times each day when you shut out phone calls and other distractions and complete a few priority chores, be it organizing your office or closet, sifting through your in-box, catching up on correspondence, or other tasks. The sense of having made some headway on finishing one or more tasks can make a person feel less pressured to catch up later by multitasking.

Multitasking often sneaks up on us, and even though we think we are getting a lot done, we may be operating less efficiently and can become disorganized. To combat this problem, try to put aside all but the most important task and complete it before moving on. You can also try making a list of your tasks and either complete them one-by-one in order of importance, or simply assign yourself particular tasks at certain times throughout the day. With practice, most people can become more aware of when they begin and finish a task, making them less likely to take on multiple duties simultaneously.

The Power of "No"

"No"—it's often a child's favorite word, yet many adults have a hard time saying it. When we use the word effectively, it can go a long way toward lowering stress levels.

When people don't say "no" enough, they can find themselves taking on too many responsibilities. They may then feel anxious, resentful, and perhaps a little bit "trapped" by all the tasks they have committed to but cannot possibly complete. Even requests that seem minor at first, or are set way in the future, eventually roll around and have to be piled on to one's list of responsibilities and tasks. Because time is a limited commodity for many of us, agreeing to do too many favors, chair another luncheon, be on another committee, volunteer for yet another cause, or even give someone a ride to an appointment can sometimes become overwhelming and a major source of stress.

At seventy-three, Anna, Shirley's mother, was the adored matriarch of the family. Throughout her life, she had always taken care of everyone, and hadn't stopped yet. Although she had been a straight-A student in high school and could have gone on to any college she chose, Anna instead took a job as a secretary to support her new husband through business school. She single-handedly reared their four children without the nannies and the maids that her own kids seemed to require for *their* children. If one of her grandkids ever wanted a special something, whether it was a snack, a CD, or the hottest new toy, she raced to at least three stores until she found the right item or at least brought back an assortment for them to choose from.

Anna cultivated an image of herself as the ultimate earth mother—she prided herself on helping others and had a terrible time turning down any request from her family and friends. But lately, Anna seemed irritable, and it seemed to her family that she resented doing some of the things she did. Perhaps driving her husband, Frank, everywhere since he had developed phlebitis and caring for her sister who had Alzheimer's was becoming too much for her, with all her other self-imposed duties.

Anna wasn't big on asking for help, either, much to the exasperation of her daughters. When her youngest, Shirley, asked what she could bring to Thanksgiving dinner, Anna responded, "Oh, you don't need to do that, dear."

"But, Mom, I really want to bring something to help out," Shirley insisted. "How about some dessert? I'll stop by the bakery on my way up, okay?"

"Oh, honey, I don't want you to spend any money, but if you insist, just bring anything you want . . . Maybe your chopped cucumber salad . . . or your homemade bread, but please no raisins or nuts in it. You know how Daddy is."

The family knew that something was seriously wrong when Shirley got to her mother's home on Thanksgiving. She walked into the kitchen with the cucumber salad and a store-bought loaf of crusty French bread, and said hello to her mom, sister, and her two sisters-in-law. Suddenly, in front of them all, Anna grabbed the salad plate from Shirley and threw it on the floor, yelling, "You couldn't even *make* the bread?! I've been slaving all week, *and* taking care of your aunt and your father, and not one of you girls even *offered* to have Thanksgiving at your house!" Anna stormed out of the room sobbing, leaving the others stunned.

For people like Anna, saying "no" contradicts their perception of who they are, just as asking for help might never enter their minds. Anna was unable to gauge when the expectations she had put on herself had become unrealistic. This led her to feel a sense of desperation, and her difficulty in asking for help only made it worse. After her family convinced her to see a psychotherapist, Anna became more aware of her own needs, which helped her to say no when the requests of others were just not reasonable for her to fulfill. She also got into a support group for caregivers of Alzheimer's patients and enlisted her children's help with driving her husband around.

Often, learning to take better care of ourselves increases our enjoyment in assisting others. To help you feel more comfortable saying "no" when it makes sense, try some of the following strategies.

The upside of "no." Keep in mind that when you say no to a request, you are saying yes to something else. Not taking on the extra assignment at work will give you more time to enjoy the weekend with your family.

Make the rules and keep them. If a friend or colleague asks for a loan or favor that makes you uncomfortable, you might try telling them that "as a rule" you don't loan money to friends, help people move, and so on. This minimizes potentially hurtful feelings and may save your friendship or work relationship. This "as a rule" technique also works well with teenagers who tend to repeat the same requests often. You can eventually resort to merely saying, "You know the rule . . ."

Ignore pressure. If you're not sure about how to respond to a request, stall. Politely tell the requester that you'll get back to them after checking your schedule. That way, you can take more time to weigh the pros and cons of the request. If you are being pressured for a decision at that very moment, then you could simply deny the request due to the decision-making time constraint.

Be straightforward. Everyone gets busy from time to time, be it scrambling to meet a work deadline, planning an event, or caring for a sick friend or family member. Sometimes it can become stressful to keep commitments we've already made, and being straightforward about the situation is often the best approach. Most people can empathize with being overcommitted and can usually find an alternate solution.

A Mad, Mad World

Anger is a common and sometimes healthy response to stressful situations. People frequently report experiencing a sense of relief after getting their angry feelings "off their chest," and sometimes a reasonable expression of anger can lead to the resolution of a stressful situation. Neuroscientists recently pinpointed a specific brain region that is stimulated when people get insulted and prepare to exact revenge. This is the same area of the brain that gets stimulated when people prepare to satisfy hunger and other cravings—mostly pleasurable. This research backs up the idea that "revenge is sweet." However, just as a very hungry person may overeat at a buffet, a person who feels wronged may occasionally overindulge in their payback. Sometimes forgiveness and empathy can help an angry person rise above his or her desire for revenge, and this is almost always the best path to a peaceful resolution (also see Essential 3).

When we get angry, we can also get upset, and uncontrolled anger can lead to rage, hostility, and unhappiness. People who get angry quickly with little or no provocation may actually have a shorter life expectancy. Expressing anger arouses the nervous system and can increase heart rate, blood pressure, and risk for strokes. There is also evidence that people with an angry temperament have a greater risk for heart disease.

Holding our anger inside is not the answer, either. People who hold in their emotions and suffer silently tend to have higher stress hormone levels than those with healthy anger outlets. Systematic studies point to an optimal, intermediate level of anger expression, somewhere between unbridled outbursts and complete containment. In that way, we are able to modulate the stress hormone release that accompanies controlled anger expressions without blowing our tops, and perhaps saying things we can't take back.

There are various approaches to managing anger. Most techniques are aimed at helping people become aware of their underlying triggers, learn to control their angry feelings, and use relaxation techniques to minimize their physical responses to those feelings. Uncontrollable anger can sometimes be a symptom of another problem, such as depression, excessive drinking, or drug abuse. Regardless of the cause of chronic temper tantrums, a person must first admit to having a problem before any approach can succeed. Almost everyone can learn how to be assertive and appropriately express anger without becoming aggressive or destructive.

Laugh in the Face of Stress

Everyone likes a good laugh. Humor allows us to release tension and let go of fearful or angry feelings, even if just for a little while. Norman Cousins was a champion of using humor to battle his painful and crippling arthritic disease, and systematic research has supported such health-promoting effects of humor.

Japanese scientists recently studied a group of volunteers who watched a popular comedy show while dining, and compared them to another group eating the same meal but watching a boring lecture (not mine, I swear). After dinner, the group that laughed more had more stable blood sugar levels, and stability of blood sugar is known to lower the risk for diabetes.

Laughter may protect us against heart disease, as well. In a recent study of three hundred volunteers, scientists found that the people *without* heart disease were 60 percent more likely to see humor in everyday life. Other studies have linked watching a daily half-hour sitcom with lower blood pressure and improved heartbeat regularity, both of which lower risk for heart attacks.

Apparently, just anticipating a humorous situation has health benefits. Volunteers who were told that they would see a favorite comic in three days had a drop in their stress hormone levels and a boost in levels of chemicals that strengthen the immune system. Other research has found that laughter improves our ability to tolerate pain. Whether you prefer old W. C. Fields movies, hanging out at comedy clubs, or simply reading the Sunday funnies, a regular dose of laughter may not only lift your spirits but bolster your longevity.

Muscle Relaxation Exercise:
Wind Up and Unwind

Do this lying down or in a comfortable chair. While the rest of your body remains comfortable and relaxed, slowly clench your right fist as tightly as you can. Focus on the tension in your right fist, hand, and forearm. After five seconds, relax your hand, let your fingers and wrist go limp, and relax for fifteen to thirty seconds. Notice the sensations of tension and relaxation in those muscles. Now repeat with your left fist, then relax. Next, bend your right elbow, tense your biceps muscle, and hold that tension for five seconds. Then let your arm straighten and drop gently to your side and relax for fifteen to thirty seconds. Repeat the exercise for your left side. Continue this sequence of tensing and releasing different muscle groups sequentially up your arms, through your shoulders, chest, face, back, abdomen, buttocks, legs, and feet. After you have completed moving through to your toes, tense your entire body for five seconds and then fully relax. Take several deep breaths and savor the feeling of muscle relaxation.

Sleep On It

An estimated 100 million Americans suffer from the stress of insomnia, which can cause memory impairment, fatigue, irritability, and a variety of other problems. The National Highway Traffic Safety Administration estimates that drivers falling asleep at the wheel cause more than 100,000 auto accidents each year. Cheating on your sleep may also grow your waistline. Researchers recently found that not getting enough sleep elevates blood levels of appetite-stimulating hormones and is associated with a greater risk for being overweight.

The average person needs about seven to eight hours of sleep each night, but our sleep needs decline as we age. People who are sleep deprived tend to lack energy and motivation; they often feel "fuzzy headed" or confused the next day. Although getting enough hours of sleep is a stress-reduction goal, not all sleep is equal. For sleep to be restorative, we need to *remain* asleep throughout the night. Even subtle noises that don't actually awaken us can be disruptive enough to affect the quality of our sleep. That is why falling asleep with the TV on may leave us feeling tired the next day.

The following are a few tips that can help people get the sleep they need:

- *Stay on schedule.* Our bodies naturally adjust to regular daily cycles. Sometimes sleep problems result from our schedule being temporarily out of sync with our normal lifestyle requirements. Try to get into bed the same time each evening, and set your alarm for the same time each morning. To keep your body on its routine, don't sleep too late on the weekends and avoid napping during the day.
- *Quiet down before bedtime.* Once in bed, try avoiding TV or eating. If you read, try to skip overly exciting stories that might hype you up. Those who listen to music before bed should stick with the more serene sounds and save the heavy metal for the daytime activities. Caffeine, and liquids in general, should be avoided. Also, remain mindful of when you first notice fatigue—that's the moment you want to turn out the light, get yourself in a comfortable position, and let yourself relax.
- *Take to the tub.* Many people find that a warm shower or bath before bedtime relaxes their muscles and helps them get to sleep.
- *Create a comfort zone.* Arrange the bedroom furniture, light, and sound level so they maximize calm and comfort (see Essential 5).

- *Get active during the day.* One of the best ways to sleep through the night is to make sure you get plenty of physical activity during the day. Plan your workout sessions well before bedtime so they don't leave you overenergized, which can make it difficult to relax.
- *Talk with your doctor.* Chronic insomnia may be a symptom of depression or other medical conditions, so consult your physician if your efforts at promoting sleep are ineffective.

Acupuncture: Meet the Needles

This ancient Chinese therapy has been used as a treatment for several forms of pain and a variety of stress-related conditions. During acupuncture, thin needles are inserted into the skin at specific points on the body. Some forms of acupuncture use heat, pressure, or mild electrical current to stimulate the energy at these points, instead of needles.

The Chinese theorize that *chi* energy flows through the body along pathways, or *meridians*, and blockage of this energy causes illness. Traditional practitioners believe acupuncture unblocks these pathways and balances the flow of chi, restoring health. Some Western medical practitioners suggest other explanations for how acupuncture might work. Dr. Hélène Langevin of the University of Vermont reported that acupuncture points correlate with areas of thick connective tissue, which also contain high concentrations of nerve endings. Stimulating these regions might affect nerve areas that transmit pain signals. The treatment boosts levels of endorphins, which can have analgesic effects. Acupuncture also elevates levels of the brain chemical serotonin, the body's natural antidepressant.

In a recent study of over fifteen thousand headache sufferers, those receiving a three-month course of weekly acupuncture treatments experienced significantly less pain than headache sufferers who received only conventional treatments. Other studies have found that acupuncture relieves pain and improves function in patients with arthritis, as compared with the control, nonpiercing treatments. Although not all studies have been positive, there is enough evidence to suggest that this age-old intervention has the potential to help many people suffering from various types of pain.

Growing Your Nest Egg

Since we are living longer, it's important to plan for it financially. By preparing ahead and getting the most value from our money, we may be able to alleviate much of our stress over financial concerns for the future. Research indicates that most people are not saving enough money to comfortably enjoy their retirement years. In fact, according to a recent survey done by the AARP, one in three retirees are forced back to work after they retire either because they failed to save enough to fully retire or because they suffered catastrophic losses with their investments. Only one out of every three Americans contributes to a tax-deferred savings account such as an IRA or one based at their job, like a 401(k) plan, to help with their retirement, and those who have a plan usually contribute less money than they could or should.

Neuroscientists may have a biological explanation for this phenomenon. Neuroimaging studies suggest that our brains are hardwired to prefer immediate gratification—enjoying the present versus saving for the future. Using functional MRI scanning, researchers at Princeton University studied the brain activity of volunteers making choices about different monetary reward options. They found that financial decisions involved two areas of the brain: the prefrontal cortex, a highly evolved decision-making brain region, and a primitive brain region known as the limbic system, which responds to decisions involving instant rewards. Study subjects who tended to be immediate gratifiers showed greater activity in this limbic region; therefore, their brain's predisposition for immediate gratification may cloud their long-term decision-making. Other studies have found that when given a choice, most people will put off what is difficult or painful, even if logically they know it is good for them in the long run.

Investment companies have been working to create new approaches to saving for the future to help people overcome the tendency to play now and save later. The sooner we get our financial planning in order, the less stress we will feel about the future. Here are a few strategies that may work for you.

- *Calculate your actual needs.* Getting a realistic idea of how much money you will have for retirement, based on your current saving habits, can either be a comforting stress-reliever or a wake-up call to make changes. An accountant, financial planner, or investment consultant can help you accurately calculate these figures.
- *Get tough about current spending.* Take a serious look at how you are spending your money today. While reviewing your patterns, look for an item that you pay for on a regular basis that you could possibly cut back on. It can actually be a fun challenge to try to save money by skipping an unnecessary foray to the shoe department or the makeup counter and instead, taking a nice, *free* walk in the fresh air.
- *Opt for the plan.* Employees are often presented with company savings-plan options in a way that lets inertia get the better of them—the default position is *no* plan, and people need to make an extra effort to opt *for* a plan. When companies switch from optional to automatic enrollment and people must opt *out* instead of opt *in* to a plan, there are dramatic in-

creases in the proportion of people who put some of their money away for retirement.

- *Push yourself*. If you are currently contributing one percent of your earnings to a 401(k), try to notch it up to two or three percent—you may not even feel the pinch too badly. The next time you get a raise or your expenses go down, seize the opportunity to sock away more for retirement.

- *Make your contributions automatic*. That way you don't have to think about contributing at regular intervals. With future savings, out of sight means out of your hands to spend now. Whether or not your work has a retirement plan available, there are several other mechanisms you can use, such as IRAs or savings bonds purchase plans. A professional financial planner can help you choose one that meets your needs.

- *Keep an eye on your investments*. Saving and investing is an excellent start, but you also have to avoid taking undue risk with your investments. Suffering capital losses can create financial and emotional stress. Most financial advisors recommend avoiding risky investments as people approach retirement age.

Workplace Stress

People rarely do their best work under pressure, yet almost everyone has experienced stress at work at some point. Stress on the job can have a major impact on our health and well-being. Workplace stress can come from a variety of sources, including relationships, unrealistic job expectations, and even the actual physical workplace environment (see Essential 5).

Stress arising directly from an issue with the boss has been found to negatively affect the employee's health. Scientists recently found that when health care personnel worked for a boss they thought was unfair, their systolic blood pressure (when the heart contracts) increased by thirteen points and diastolic (between contractions) increased by six points on average. That's enough to increase risk for a stroke by nearly 40 percent. When the employees worked for a boss whom they respected and trusted, one who supported them with praise and feedback, the workers' blood pressure actually decreased slightly.

Other studies have found that the risk of dying from a heart attack doubles among employees during times of major company downsizing. One analysis of more than twenty-four thousand Swedish workers found that during periods of large-scale mergers, workers were more likely to take sick leave or to go to the hospital because of illness.

Much of an employee's stress on the job appears to arise from the combination of high job demands and a limited sense of control. When people feel they do have some control in their workplace—a sense of power to direct their own actions—they feel more satisfied, experience less stress, and have better health outcomes. Because we are often unable to eliminate the source of our workplace stress, finding other ways to relax can help us avoid some of the negative physical and emotional consequences.

- *Organize and avoid procrastination.* At the start of each day, spend a few minutes setting priorities and organizing the day ahead. Be realistic about what you can accomplish and avoid putting off difficult tasks. Making this a regular morning habit can help anchor you and keep you focused. It also helps minimize multitasking.
- *Fine-tune your communication skills.* One of the greatest sources of workplace stress can be communication problems and misunderstandings. Try to be specific in formulating questions or complaints and avoid getting into conflicts that

do not directly involve you. When conflicts do arise, listen carefully before explaining your own position. If possible, don't involve your superiors in a conflict with a colleague unless your own attempts to work it out have failed. Keep in mind that everything you put in writing—particularly e-mail—can become a permanent, public record, so choose your written words wisely.

• *Cool it on the caffeine.* Though modest amounts of caffeine can increase alertness, too much leads to irritability and anxiety, which only adds to stress. Avoid running to the coffeepot when the pressure is on.

• *Take regular stretching and relaxation breaks.* Get up and stretch or do a breathing exercise at regular intervals. If possible, try going outdoors or opening a window to get some fresh air during work breaks. Set your watch alarm to remind you to stretch and move around. Relaxing your muscles throughout the day is a preemptive strike against stress.

• *Delegate.* People who have a hard time delegating often feel unnecessarily stressed-out. Asking people to help you by doing tasks that they can handle allows you more time to complete the work that perhaps only you can do.

• *Adapt your personal environment.* Photos and other personal items add character and a homey feeling to your workspace, which can contribute to a sense of calm. To increase comfort and avoid injury, read up on workplace ergonomic principles (see Essential 5). Sometimes simply adjusting the angle of your chair and the position of your keyboard, or perhaps propping your feet up on a box, can ease muscle tension and reduce stress.

• *Power nap.* For people who are behind on their sleep, a few winks in the afternoon can often make them more alert and energetic throughout the rest of the day. A recent study of volunteers who were allowed to nap for thirty minutes demonstrated that they had greater job productivity afterward, as compared with those who did not nap (see box).

Tips for Effective Power Napping

1. Limit your nap to no more than thirty minutes. Longer naps generally leave us feeling tired and groggy. Aim for the twenty-minute power nap.
2. Many people avoid daytime napping because they fear they will oversleep. Use a timer or alarm so that won't happen.
3. People with private offices only need to close the door and turn off the phone to get some quiet time. Those with more public workspaces may need to be creative in finding a quiet, private spot. Some people like to nap in their car or a shady spot in a park during their lunch break.
4. Don't worry if you cannot fall asleep. Just relaxing with your eyes closed can help you to feel more rested after nap time.

More Proven Stress Busters

There are a variety of other approaches that not only reduce stress, but also improve fitness, balance, and mental clarity. The following list includes a few examples.

- *Yoga.* This ancient Indian practice promotes health and relaxation through a sequence of physical poses and breathing exercises that build strength, balance, and flexibility. It is effective in reducing stress and increasing mental clarity. Yoga has also been found to lower cholesterol levels and blood pressure, and a recent scientific study found that yoga combined with meditation in a six-week stress-reduction program led to significant improvements in cardiac health.

- *Tai chi.* Pronounced *"tie-chee,"* this Chinese form of exercise can reduce stress, increase strength, improve balance, and help prevent falls in seniors. Many of the movements, originally derived from martial arts, are performed slowly and gracefully, and emphasize deep breathing and relaxation. Scientists recently found that tai chi can improve heart and lung function. Researchers at the Semel Institute for Neuroscience and Human Behavior at UCLA reported that fifteen weeks of tai chi helped protect older adults against the shingles virus (the same virus that causes chickenpox), suggesting that the practice may boost immune function. Chi gong (pronounced *"chee-gong"*) is a related ancient Chinese practice that shares many similar exercises that improve mental focus, movement, and breathing.

- *Self-hypnosis.* This method generally combines relaxation techniques with visualization and imagery to induce a hypnotic state, which is essentially a very deep form of relaxation. Self-hypnosis has been found to lower stress levels, reduce pain, and alleviate some allergy symptoms. It can also improve concentration and memory ability.

- *Massage.* Besides reducing stress, massage therapy has been used to relieve symptoms of various conditions, including migraine headache, back and neck pain, and fibromyalgia. Some experts speculate that massage may do more than just provide temporary pain relief and may actually activate the body's immune system. The National Institutes of Health has a Center for Complementary and Alternative Medicine that is pursuing systematic studies on the health benefits of massage, and initial results are encouraging.

- *Get active and social.* Physical activity not only improves health and strength, but helps us relax—partly due to the hormone endorphin—the natural antidepressant our bodies secrete during aerobic exercise. Enjoying a game of tennis or a brisk walk with a friend may reduce stress through the emotional benefits of social interaction.

- *Control clutter.* Many people are unaware that a disorganized, overly cluttered home, work space, kitchen, closet, or any other place in which we spend time can lead to stress and heightened levels of the stress hormone cortisol. Reducing the clutter around us is a lifelong challenge that is best handled on a daily basis—by putting things where they belong and tossing anything we don't need—before clutter gets out of hand (see Essential 5).

- *Open up.* One of the most effective ways to reduce stress is to talk about feelings with someone you trust. Whether it's your spouse, a best friend, or a professional, getting things off your chest can often help put problems into perspective and detoxify a stressful situation.

- *Plan ahead.* Sometimes we know about or can anticipate a stressful situation before it occurs. It may be an upcoming holiday dinner at the home of a relative who always insults you, or having to show up at work Monday morning and report to an underling who got *your* promotion. Try looking at these situations as *advance notices*—opportunities to arm ourselves emotionally to cope with the stress, and possibly avoid repeating mistakes we've made in similar situations when we didn't have time to prepare. Of course, whenever feasible, simply steering clear of a stressful situation altogether is a good longevity choice, but in many cases it just isn't possible.

Because everyone will respond differently to the various stress-reduction techniques available, it's a good idea to try several approaches until you find one or more that works best. Documented evidence shows that many of these techniques not only help you relax, but will benefit your health and longevity as well.

Living Stress Free

- Practice mindful awareness—staying in the moment and being aware of what is going on inside your body—through meditation, relaxation techniques, yoga, or other exercises you enjoy. Take stress release breaks throughout the day.
- Avoid multitasking by scheduling a regular time each day for completing priority chores; try finishing one task before beginning another.
- Learn to say "no" when you need to.
- Modulate stress with healthy expressions of anger.
- Use humor to gain perspective on stressful situations.
- Get a good night's sleep every night. Take simple steps to beat insomnia without medication.
- Discover ways to limit stress on the job.
- Place emphasis on saving for the future.
- Reduce stress by decluttering your personal environment.
- Plan your strategy for dealing with stressful events you know about in advance.

Essential 5

Master Your Environment

It isn't pollution that's harming the environment. It's the impurities in our air and water that are doing it.

— DAN QUAYLE

Barbara W. brought cookies and tea up to her husband Greg's study as he worked late on a case he was trying in the morning. He had to shift two large piles of papers and a stack of legal files, but still knocked the phone and a tray of correspondence off his massive desk just to make room for the teacup. Barbara anxiously helped him pick up the papers. She always hated coming into this room—the crazy, cluttered disarray of binders, folders, documents, and scribbled notes made her skin crawl. "How can you work in this mess?" she asked him for the millionth time. He shrugged. "I know, I know, as soon as I close these two cases, I'm going to clean up in here and organize things." He relaxed back in his chair, propped his feet on another pile of files, and returned to work.

The next night, Barbara cleared the dinner dishes as Greg excused himself to his study. Twenty seconds later he shrieked, "Barbara!" She came running in to find him standing in the center of his now clean, organized, glistening study—files all tucked in the drawers and the desk polished and clear—with phone, computer, and fax machine neatly arranged on its surface. "What the hell happened?!" he demanded. "You like it?" she asked excitedly. "Maria and I cleaned up in here today." Panicked, he rifled through the desk. "Where's the Mitchelson file?! I can't find the Mitchelson file!" Barbara went to the file cabinets. "I'll help you find it." "No!" he yelled. "You've already wrecked my entire organizational system! The Mitchelson file was on top of the third pile from the left, behind the phone, next to the fax machine! It had two yellow paper clips!"

Our environment, everything around us, directly influences not just how we feel, but also how well we function and how long we live. The places where we reside, work, and play affect us both physically and emotionally—and each of us responds differently to various environmental factors. Whether it's features of the environment at large, such as traffic, noise, and smog, or more personal environmental issues, such as clutter, smoke, or aesthetics, our quality longevity requires that we adapt to these influences, or *adapt them*, to meet our individual needs.

Aesthetic Living

When creating a comfortable home or work environment, we need to focus on function *and* the emotional impact of the space. Everyone has his or her own tastes in style and aesthetics; successful interior designers often get to know their clients personally in order to be able to evoke certain feelings in the rooms they design for them.

A sparsely decorated, modern living room may instantly relax one person, whereas a shabby chic/country decor may be just the ticket to make another person feel cozy and at home. Choices of art and color can generate an atmosphere that enhances or detracts from our emotional state. A warm color like red might alert one person to danger, while for another it evokes passion. Blues, greens, and neutral browns often produce a calming ambience.

A popular approach to home decorating, feng shui (pronounced *"fung schway"*), is the ancient Chinese art of arranging home or work environments to promote health, happiness, and prosperity. Feng shui consultants advise their clients on many details of their surroundings—from color choices to furniture placement.

Although feng shui is unfamiliar to some Westerners, many of its recommendations utilize common sense to enhance environments. One principle takes note of the importance of one's first impression upon entering a home. Creating a warm and welcoming feeling may be as simple as placing a large vase of flowers in the corner of the entry room. Also, moving beds, desks, and couches from under any overhead beams can help to avoid the feeling that something is "hanging over you." For cramped spaces, a feng shui expert may recommend hanging mirrors and eliminating any unnecessary furniture to create the impression of roominess.

The sounds and noises around us, as well as the music we listen to, have an important impact on our mood and quality of life. Listening to music has been found to increase surgeons' speed and accuracy during their procedures. A specific type of sound, in a process known as vibroacoustic therapy, has been used to reduce stress and pain symptoms. Listening to classical music has been found to lower stress-related elevations in blood pressure, and individual music choices, whether it's country music, rock, or rap, may improve mood and quality of life. Fountains or other water treatments are soothing to the ear, visually calming, and effective at masking annoying traffic sounds.

Surrounding ourselves with artwork, appealing textures, and comfortable furniture not only adds to the warmth of our environment, it also helps to lower stress and give us a sense of sanctuary. Displaying photos and gifts from people we love will help to remind us of their presence. Natural light and plants, as well as areas for quiet time and reflection, indoors and outdoors, all contribute to the aesthetics and function of our surroundings.

The Bedroom: The Final Frontier

We spend nearly one third of our lives sleeping. The way in which we arrange our bedroom environment can foster or hinder the sense of security and comfort that helps us get to sleep. The amount of sleep we get each night has a much greater impact on our health and quality longevity than many of us realize.

Although not getting enough sleep has health risks, getting too much sleep may be harmful as well. In a survey of more than 100,000 people, Japanese scientists recently found that people who slept eight or more hours each night had higher mortality rates compared with those sleeping only seven hours. However, sleeping less than four and a half hours was found to increase mortality risks as well.

Sleep also affects appetite. When we don't get enough sleep, our bodies produce inadequate amounts of a hormone that helps us to feel sated after we eat, so lack of sleep can actually lead to increased appetite and weight gain. For most people, somewhere between six and seven hours of sleep each night is associated with good health and quality longevity.

To help ensure a restful and peaceful sleep setting, pay attention to some of the following details:

Mattresses. You may swear by a certain mattress, while your partner swears *at* it. Perhaps the most important consideration in choosing a mattress is to test several different ones and determine what feels right, keeping in mind both comfort and firmness. Encasing the mattress with an allergen-blocking cover will protect you against small particles and dust mites.

Bedding. High-count cotton linens tend to be softer, making it easier for many people to fall and stay asleep. Thread-counts can range anywhere from two hundred to eight hundred, but the extremely fine sheets (those with higher thread-counts) are more expensive and tend to fall apart or need replacement after repeated washings. Your pillow choice is important, as well. Wool or goose down pillows may provide more contoured neck and shoulder support, but people with allergies might do better with a molded foam pillow. Keep in mind that even synthetic pillows can harbor dust mites. The best protection is an allergen-blocking cover. Also, for people with low-back pain, an additional pillow under the knees (for people who sleep face up) or between the knees (for side sleepers) helps to reduce muscle strain and improve comfort levels.

Lighting. If you enjoy reading in bed, be sure you have enough illumination to avoid eyestrain or headache, although not *too* much lighting, because glaring high-wattage may not be conducive to helping you drift off to a restful night's sleep. If your bedroom gets direct sun exposure in the mornings, consider window treatments that block the light if you don't want to awaken too early. When you do get up, be sure to let sunlight into the room. This is a great way to start the day and can protect against seasonal mood swings or winter depression.

Noise and temperature. Take into account noise that might awaken you, whether it's the roadside traffic, a barking dog, or a snoring spouse. Excessive snoring might be a symptom of sleep apnea, an often treatable condition. For other unavoidable noises, try ear plugs or a "white noise" machine that plays waves or other calming sounds. Make sure that your wake-up alarm is gentle, rather than shrill or high-pitched. You might try soothing music to help start your day off right.

Most people prefer a comfortably cool room for sleeping, approximately sixty-five to sixty-seven degrees Fahrenheit, allowing one or more blankets to give warmth and coziness to the bed. Try opening a window, using a fan on a low setting, or, if the weather demands it, air-conditioning or heating.

Reading and TV. Experts suggest winding down with an enjoyable, relaxing activity during the hour before bedtime. It is best to avoid watching exciting television shows or reading thriller-type books during that period because they may stimulate you instead of the opposite. If TV helps you to nod off, attempt to use an automatic shut-off button so you won't be awakened in the middle of the night by a blaring infomercial. Insomniacs often do best by eliminating TV from the bedroom altogether.

Clutter Control

Often it's subtle: You walk into a room and begin to feel uneasy, confused, or edgy—yet you haven't a clue why. The next time this happens, scan your surroundings. You may be suffering from clutter overload—the psychological effects of a disorganized, overly packed room, home, closet, or work space.

Scientists have found that laboratory animals in crowded, cluttered cages become ornery, agitated, and antisocial. Chronic crowding, clutter, and disorganization can lead to high levels of the stress hormone cortisol, which can impair memory and concentration and aggravate a wide range of age-related diseases.

Reducing clutter and maintaining an organized home and work space is a lifelong daily challenge. Typically we come home after a busy day, grab the mail, maybe drag in some packages, and never get around to putting everything away—a stack of magazines and junk mail stays on the counter, a jacket gets draped on a chair instead of hung in the closet, and so on. There's also a tendency to surround ourselves with papers, computer accessories, files, photographs, CDs, clothes, books, laundry, dishes, magazines, and more. Over time, clutter may build up until we can no longer find what we need. Some people would rather drive to the hardware store and buy a new screwdriver than dig through the garage to find the one they know they have buried somewhere.

In its extreme, clutter can escalate to pathological levels. We've all heard of those "pack rats" that cannot help but collect old newspapers, magazines, or clothes to the point that their personal clutter overtakes their surroundings. This form of obsessive-compulsive disorder can be treated professionally, but many clutter junkies adamantly resist letting go of their precious collections.

Most of us, thankfully, can easily manage our surroundings by using some of the following clutter-control tips.

- *Think small.* Reorganize and declutter one room or area of that room at a time. Trying to take on the entire house or office is overwhelming and reduces the likelihood that you'll stay with the task.
- *Box it.* Separate items and place them into one of three boxes: Designate one as a *donation* box, a second for *things to keep*, and a third as the *uncertain* collection. Use these same boxes for each area of your home or office that you tackle.
- *Let things go.* Get your "donation" box items out of the house ASAP. Next, go through your "uncertain" box—if you haven't

used something in the last twelve months, move the item to the donation box now—no whining.

- *Sort now.* When you receive mail or bring in groceries, sort them right away. For junk mail, try returning the postage-paid envelope with a note asking to be removed from the mailing list.
- *Arrange by similarities.* Take your "keep" piles and search for similarities among items, whether by function, color, or texture. Organize and put away these similar items together, so they will be easy to find later. It will be much easier to find the key to the gate padlock if it's in the designated key box, rather than "somewhere in one of the kitchen drawers." Labeling the key would be helpful, as well.
- *Put away rarely used items.* Your ski clothes don't need a prominent position in your closet during the summer months. Rarely used or seasonal items should be stored in less frequented places, such as a spare bedroom closet or attic.
- *Isolate necessary clutter.* None of us can entirely remove all the clutter from our lives, but we can reserve smaller spaces for clutter control. Whether it's a classic "junk drawer" in the kitchen, a closet in that extra bedroom, or a box in the attic, make sure it's an area that is out of sight. Also, sift through the isolated clutter at regular intervals and dispose of things, especially if the clutter is filling up that area or becoming unmanageable.
- *Schedule declutter time.* Train yourself to spend five to ten minutes each day to sort through any gathering clutter. Carry a paper bag around the house and scan your major living spaces. Are books, magazines, or mail beginning to pile up? Is your closet, desk, or pantry becoming disorganized? Sorting and tossing a bit each day helps you avoid the need for organization marathons.

Information Overload: Managing Technology

Over the last few decades, technological developments in computers, telecommunications, and more have transformed our environments. Futurists predict that soon we will be able to exchange video calls as commonly as e-mail. Everything from tracking medical records to operating home appliances to making dinner reservations will be carried out by our rapidly emerging global networks.

What we're seeing is an explosion of information technology, and our computers are becoming not just more enjoyable but also more useful. Even psychotherapy is available online. At a recent conference sponsored by the U.S. Department of Health and Human Services, scientists reported that "talk therapy" delivered via the Internet on hand-held organizers was effective in treating patients with anxiety and social phobia. However, recent studies suggest that automation advances are often coupled with inefficiencies. With increasingly complex programs, we are seeing more software glitches and computer crashes that waste time and reduce productivity.

The resulting information overload is creating a new form of clutter mania. Computer desktops and file systems collect clutter as much as our jam-packed closets and drawers. It's not just electronic data, but hard copies, as well. The average American consumes more than two tons of paper each year.

We're choking on information to the point of exhaustion, from electronic billboards, cell phones, radio, cable, satellite TV with ticker-tape headlines, and even plasma screens in elevators. A current *New York Times* Sunday edition probably contains more information than the average person was ever exposed to during their lifetime just one hundred years ago. Faced with too much information, we can become desensitized, indecisive, and frustrated.

Some concerns about this new technology, however, appear to be myths more than actual risks. For example, a popular urban legend has it that overuse of cell phones can cause brain tumors. A group of Danish epidemiologists systematically investigated this question and failed to confirm that cellular phone use had any effect on the incidence or size of brain tumors.

It is estimated that 75 percent of young adults and 20 percent of seniors use the Internet, with use among seniors jumping dramatically during the past decade. One of the greatest incentives for their Internet use is staying in touch with family members. Younger family members encourage their parents and grandparents to set up e-mail accounts, and the older folks love it. Several resources are available on the Internet to help seniors develop their Internet skills, including *www.generationsonline.com* and *www.seniornet.org.*

It is estimated that more than 60 percent of all e-mail users check their e-mail once a day and one third of users check it several times a day. The rise in popularity of instant messaging and handheld Internet devices, such as the BlackBerry, have turned some people into virtual e-mail addicts — remaining immersed in online chatter for hours at a time. Though the quick and easy exchange of electronic information is efficient, too much technology use causes some people to disconnect from face-to-face human contact. E-mail tends to have an informal quality to it, which can lower our inhibitions when communicating. Without in-person visual cues, it is easier to misinterpret what gets said. Interoffice e-mails have become so problematic that many businesses are now legally obligated to monitor them.

Joyce and Brian carried the large, wrapped box into her parents' house, and the kids followed carrying a birthday cake and card. Joyce's mom, Ellen, was seventy today, and they all gathered around as she opened her present—a brand-new personal computer. Ellen smiled, a little disappointed. "You guys, really, you shouldn't have spent so much. I'll never learn to use this thing. And Daddy won't touch it—unless it's made of chocolate." Grandpa chuckled—she got that right. He was still figuring out how to use the remote control for the new TV they gave him last Christmas.

Ignoring her protests, Joyce told Brian to set the computer up in the den. "Don't worry, Mom, you're going to love it. You can e-mail the kids, see pictures of them, find new recipes, play bridge, all kinds of things. And we already signed you up for an online service."

With Joyce's help, Ellen learned how to use the computer, and started e-mailing with the kids once or twice a week. She shared photographs of her grandchildren with friends over the Web, and she liked trading cooking tips and recipes in a chat room that Joyce helped her find.

Two weeks later, Joyce slammed down the telephone receiver as Brian came home from work. "Whoa, what's going on?" Joyce went back to making dinner. "My folks' line has been busy for three hours!" Brian gave her a kiss. "It's probably just off the hook, honey. I'm sure everything's fine."

Another month went by and the kids hadn't seen their grandparents in weeks. Joyce called her mom about getting together. "But Sunday is Father's Day and we *always* come over." She listened. "Let me speak to Daddy." She paused. "Okay, fine. We'll be there Sunday at four. Bye."

When they arrived at the folks' place on Sunday, Grandpa was watching a ball game in the living room. The house was a mess—dishes, glasses, soda cans, and unfolded laundry were everywhere, and even Grandpa himself hadn't shaved. Ellen was in the den, on the computer. Joyce approached her. "Mom?" "Not now!" Ellen hissed. "I'm up $500!" Joyce, horrified, saw that her mother was playing Internet poker.

Joyce and Brian sent the kids outside to play and had a serious talk with the folks. Apparently, Ellen had begun Internet gambling some weeks ago, and unbeknownst to Grandpa, she had developed a little "habit"—to the tune of a $3,500 loss. Unfortunately, other losses—her relationships with her husband, friends, and family—were just becoming apparent. Ellen was embarrassed and not quite sure how it had taken hold of her so quickly. She promised to stop the gambling and give up her Internet use until she could get some help for her new "problem."

Ellen went to see a therapist and realized that she had to completely lock out all gambling Internet sites if she wanted to keep the computer, because she had become addicted. He encouraged her to join a twelve-step program for gamblers. Her husband, friends, and family kept an eye on her and encouraged her to keep off the gambling sites. And it wasn't really hard to do—she was far too busy now bidding for really great things on eBay. She hadn't mentioned that to her therapist yet.

Computers were designed to enhance our daily lives, not to overtake them. Just as we can control the foods we eat, we can monitor and limit the amount of information we take in, preventing it from bombarding us and eroding the limited time we have to spend with important people in our lives. The following are some simple steps we can take to reduce the fatigue, confusion, and stress of too much technology and information.

- *Protect your address.* Anyone who uses e-mail or the Internet knows how easy it is to wind up on those mass-market spam e-mail lists. If you find yourself getting lots of junk e-mail, scan your messages and quickly discard those that are not important. You can remove yourself from junk e-mail lists by contacting the Internet provider of the sender (*postmaster @provider-name.com*). Also, take a few minutes to download a spam filter, as well as to install spyware and virus protection software on your computer. Maintaining an unlisted telephone number will also cut down on those intrusive solicitation calls during dinner hour.

- *Just say no to newsgroups.* Unless you prefer this format for news updates, try declining newsgroup invitations in order to save time and cut down on data redundancy. Chances are you're getting the same information from newspapers, magazines, or the TV news.

- *Don't get lost on the Web.* With an estimated two billion Web pages out there, it's easy to become overwhelmed by information. Mastering some basic search techniques (see *www.metacrawler.com*) can help reduce a possible ten thousand entries to a reasonable ten.

- *Cut down on paper.* Judicious use of the printer can make a key bit of information more accessible, but paper clutter can pile up in no time at all. Any papers you don't need should be filed in the recycle bin.

- *Limit phone time.* Turn off your cell phone and hold calls during important meetings. If you must be available to some people at all times, try getting a pager and limit the access to it.

- *Get organized.* Use a file system to sort information coming in from that going out. Keep your "in" and "out" files in a convenient place on a desk or tabletop.

- *Quash junk mail.* If you contact the Direct Marketing Association (1120 Avenue of the Americas, New York, NY 10036-6700, 212-768-7277; *www.the-dma.org*), you can have your address taken off those annoying lists that lead to piles of junk mail.

TV Addiction

Television, as a tool for disseminating information, has transformed our environments—influencing our behaviors, tastes, activities, and even our beverage choices. It is among the most significant of technological tools in shaping social and political life. But one can get too much of a good thing. On average, Americans spend approximately three hours each day watching TV—more time than any other activity, except for work and sleep. Add up the total number of hours spent in front of the tube over a lifetime, and by age seventy-five it comes to *nine years*.

One reason people are drawn to watching television is that it appears to trigger an instinctive orienting response first described by Dr. Ivan Pavlov, famous for his work with dogs in the area of conditioned response. We instinctively react to the TV's novel and sudden stimuli: heart rate slows, brain blood vessels dilate, and blood flows away from major muscles. This physiological reaction helps the brain focus on the mental stimulus. Television programs typically have rapid cuts and edits, which can stimulate and maintain our attention. However, when these cuts become too frequent, they can shift our orienting response into overdrive—we continue to watch, but experience fatigue, rather than mental stimulation.

Dr. Robert Kubey of Rutgers University and Dr. Mihaly Csikszentmihalyi of Claremont Graduate University have found that prolonged TV exposure may pose hidden hazards. By systematically monitoring mood and mental states during television viewing, they found that people feel relaxed and passive while watching TV, but their level of mental stimulation is lower compared with other activities such as reading.

The researchers also found that when people stop watching television, their sense of relaxation rapidly declines, and they feel less alert. Concentration abilities diminish, and many report a sense of depletion—as if the energy has been "sucked out of them" following a TV marathon. The more people watch TV, the less they seem to enjoy it. TV addicts are quicker to experience boredom and have more difficulties with attention. They also have a greater risk for being overweight than nonaddicts.

The scientific evidence is not strong enough to start banning television altogether, and many people derive pleasure, receive information, and get other benefits from their TV viewing. Since heavy watching does have a negative impact on our psychological state, there are some simple steps we can take to better control the TV habit.

- Try planning to watch specific shows of interest with family or friends, rather than getting into the habit of just lying around for hours, channel surfing solo.
- Make a list ranking the shows you enjoy watching each week and attempt to cut out one or more at the bottom of your list.
- Consider rearranging the furniture so that the TV is not the most prominent fixture in the room. Don't let your television shape your everyday experience: Control the remote, don't let the remote control you.
- Give books a chance. Plan or set aside a reading time, perhaps before going to bed.
- Consider other activities during your usual television-watching timeslot. Try playing a game with your mate, family, or friends—see if you're still the Mahjong Maven or the King of Scrabble.

Nine-to-Five Ergonomics

Many of us spend a large proportion of time sitting at a desk. The safety and esthetics of the space around our desk affects our productivity and quality longevity. *Ergonomics* is the science of designing objects, systems, and environments so that the job fits the person. An ergonomically designed work area takes into account anatomy, physiology, and psychology, so that the environment is comfortable, safe, and efficient for its users. Proper light, posture, and positioning will minimize work-related injuries, such as back and neck pain, hand injury, eye strain, and headache.

Because a computer monitor may cause eye strain or fatigue, screen images need to appear stable and free of distortion, flicker, or jitter. Typical ergonomic challenges involve awkward body postures, excessive repetitive movements and force, and contact stress, all of which can lead to pain, numbness, tingling, stiffness, or loss of strength. Such subtle changes as lowering your arm height or elevating your foot position may help you to avoid common work-related injuries. To ensure that your workstation is ergonomically safe, check the International Ergonomics Association Web site at *http://www.iea.cc*.

Even subtle environmental influences, such as color, can have an impact on our mood and productivity. Office workers have been found to prefer red-painted offices over white ones, and studies show that productivity is significantly greater in red offices. Other experiments indicate that memory and attention are influenced by color, as well.

Thermostat settings are also important. Many workers have heated arguments on workplace temperature settings. A recent study by Dr. Alan Hedge and associates at Cornell University found that workers at a large insurance company were more productive when the office temperature was increased from sixty-eight degrees Fahrenheit to the mid-seventies. Work output improved by 150 percent, and errors declined by 44 percent.

Workplace noise pollution can also reduce productivity and, when extreme, can permanently impair hearing. A person's risk depends on both the duration and volume level (measured in deci-bels, or db) of the sound. Normal conversation (60 db) or a ringing telephone (80 db) are in the safe range, but exposure beyond eight hours to a motorcycle or hair dryer (85 db), ambulance siren (140 db), or jet engine at takeoff (140 db) can put one at risk for hearing loss. If you are concerned about the noise level at your job, you might consider wearing hearing protectors—earplugs or earmuffs—or limiting the amount of time you spend exposed to the noise.

You Are What You Breathe

One of the advantages of living in a congested city is being able to *see* the air we breathe. Who knows what they're breathing in that clear country air? Seriously, polluted air poses many health hazards—it aggravates preexisting lung conditions such as asthma, and it can elevate blood pressure. Particularly smoggy days have been linked to increased mortality rates in U.S cities, and recent research has found that smog exposure when people are young may shorten life expectancy.

Toxic air exposure from sitting in traffic can nearly triple the risk for a heart attack. A recent study of more than nine hundred heart attack victims found that patients spent more time commut-ing the very day they suffered their heart attacks than on previous days. The risk was three times greater if they had been in a car or on public transportion during the hour before the attack, and four times greater if they had been on a bicycle. The good news is that when cities successfully reduce pollution, rates of cardiovascular ill-ness decline.

Though most city dwellers cannot completely avoid breathing smoggy air, they can take steps to reduce their exposure. One strat-egy is to try to work longer hours four days a week in order to elimi-nate one day of commuting from their work week. Closing windows and car vents will reduce exposure to outside air in heavily congested areas. Also, try to stay indoors during midday peak pollution hours, and reserve jogging, bike riding, and other outdoor activities to those times of day when air pollution is at a low point, usually early evening and morning hours.

Indoor air has its hazards, as well. Prolonged exposure to indoor dust and molds may cause or aggravate allergies or asthma. Just walking around your house or sitting down on a comfy sofa can kick up dust and mold spores, sometimes causing as much air pollution to enter one's lungs as smoking a cigarette.

Although not all forms of mold are dangerous, recent high-profile lawsuits have focused attention on the hidden dangers of some forms of household molds. Mold can not only exacerbate respiratory problems, but the unexpected physical and financial difficulties often lead to stress-related symptoms, including anxiety and depression.

Many insurance companies have stopped their coverage of mold damage after paying out billions of dollars for contaminations from toxic molds such as *Stachybotrys chartarum*. This kind of indoor mold can grow anywhere there is moisture and air—tiles, carpets, furniture, drywall, crawl spaces, and air ducts. The mold colonies sometimes look like slimy splotches and have a musty odor.

The Institute of Medicine recently warned of the public health dangers posed by excessive dampness in buildings and the mold that it causes. To maintain a safe indoor air environment, keep in mind the following:

- *Inspect before you buy.* House and apartment hunting can be an emotional experience. Many people tend to go with their gut feelings about a home, which can cloud practical considerations. Invest the time and money in proper inspections to ensure that the space is environmentally safe.

- *Fix leaks.* Be vigilant about water leaks. A leaky faucet or pipe can pose a health threat, since any moisture accumulation could create a breeding site for toxic mold. Also, make sure that your home has adequate waterproofing and drainage to prevent moisture from accumulating.
- *Bite the dust.* If you are dust-sensitive, consider losing the wall-to-wall carpets, and other dust and spore collectors such as venetian blinds. Make sure you dust furniture at regular intervals with a damp cloth, and keep floors clean with a moistened mop.
- *HEPA filters.* These air systems filter out extremely small particles that worsen asthma and allergy symptoms. When purchasing a portable HEPA (high-efficiency particulate air) filter, choose one with capabilities that match the size of your room. You may need to buy more than one for several rooms or consider a central HEPA filtration system for your entire house, apartment, or workplace. Some units reduce air contamination by adding ozone to the room air, which attacks the cellular structure of bacteria and fungi.

If you feel your workplace may have mold contamination, discuss your concerns with your employer. For more information about mold or other contaminations in the workplace, check out the U.S. Department of Labor's Occupational Safety and Health Administration (OSHA) Web site (*www.osha.gov*).

Cigarettes: No Butts About It

When I was a kid, many of my friends thought that smoking was cool—they wanted to look like the Marlboro Man. Most people, even many doctors, were unaware of the health hazards of smoking. Fortunately, those hazards are much better appreciated today.

Smoking not only increases our risk for cancer, strokes, and heart disease, it even makes us *look* older. Drs. Darrick Antell and Eva Taczanoski of Columbia University studied the aging effects of smoking in thirty-four sets of identical twins age forty-five to seventy-five years. They found that the depth and severity of wrinkles, amount of excess skin, quality of skin texture, and amount of gray hair varied according to smoking history—the nonsmoking twin consistently looked younger. One twin who had smoked a pack of cigarettes every day for forty years had approximately 50 percent more gray hair than his twin brother who had never smoked. Smoking also appeared to have a much greater influence on appearance than sun exposure, exercise, diet, or alcohol use.

Once someone gets hooked on cigarettes, it can be tough to quit, but the benefits emerge rapidly after quitting. The body's carbon monoxide levels drop dramatically, and within a week, the risk of dying from a heart attack declines. Five years later, that person's heart attack risk is similar to that of someone who never smoked. Intensive counseling and educational programs, as well as nicotine patches and gum, are often effective. The antidepressant bupropion (marketed as Wellbutrin) is sometimes used to assist people in quitting smoking. Because alcohol has been found to enhance the pleasurable effects of nicotine, avoiding it may help smokers quit. Internet sites are available to help people quit, as well (*www.quit net.com*; *www.ashline.org*).

The government recently recognized the importance of smoking cessation programs by approving Medicare funding to help seniors quit smoking. The eleven-million-dollar annual cost of the Medicare program will be offset by the savings from fewer hospitalizations and health problems related to smoking.

Sunbathers Beware

Almost everyone has heard about the health risks of sunbathing; however, the sunlight that falls on our skin remains our main source of vitamin D, and scientists at Wake Forest University Baptist Medical Center recently found that exposure to ultraviolet light actually makes tanners feel more relaxed, motivating them to keep coming back for more tanning. The investigators believe that when exposed to UV light, the body secretes natural chemical endorphins, which are linked to both pain relief and feelings of euphoria.

This mood elevation may explain why people continue to tan, despite the overwhelming evidence of health risks. The sun's ultraviolet rays can damage and prematurely age the skin, cause cataracts, and suppress immune function. Prolonged unprotected sun exposure can lead to melanoma, a highly lethal cancer, if not detected and removed before it spreads.

If you do go in the sun, cover sensitive areas, wear a hat, and use a sunscreen with a Sun Protection Factor, or SPF, of fifteen or greater. The American Academy of Dermatology recommends reapplying sunscreen about every two to three hours. Also, keep in mind that ultraviolet rays will penetrate clouds and reflect off sand, water, and even concrete, so cover up and use sunscreen even on cloudy days. Try to avoid exposure during midday (generally between 10 a.m. and 4 p.m.).

Wear sunglasses that protect your eyes from ultraviolet rays. Also, check that your medications—particularly antibiotics and acne medicines—do not increase sun sensitivity. Stay away from artificial tanning devices, and examine your skin at regular intervals to make sure that there are no unusual changes. Finally, if a tan-skinned appearance is important to you, consider one of the many sunless self-tanning products available at drugstores and makeup counters.

Staying Behind the Wheel

Because we're living longer, we're seeing a larger number of older adults behind the wheel. By the year 2020, an estimated 40 million Americans age sixty-five and older will be licensed drivers. Most teenagers experience their first driver's license as a pivotal point of maturation—a time when they truly begin to feel independent and adult. The idea of relinquishing that privilege at some point is a prospect that most of us dread.

Yet as some people age, they experience a decline in reflexes, coordination, and mental acuity, which can challenge driving safety. Arthritis may limit neck flexibility, visual impairments can make it harder to spot road hazards, and as people get older they are more likely to take medicines that may interfere with mental abilities, reaction time, or memory of addresses.

Protecting environmental safety includes being realistic about the fact that some older adults pose a danger when behind the wheel. Warning signs that someone may need to recheck their driving skills include multiple accidents and/or tickets, a tendency to drive too slowly or too closely behind other cars, and a nervousness or tenuousness when making turns or other driving decisions. If in doubt, check with your local motor vehicle department or the American Automobile Association for resources to help seniors stay safe on the road. The AARP also offers a Driver Safety Program class (call 1-888-227-7669 for more information).

An easy way to start minimizing the risk of accidents is to reduce the time one spends behind the wheel. Not only has the amount of time spent driving been correlated with stress levels, it is also associated with becoming overweight. A recent study found that for every additional half hour in the car, the risk for obesity increases by 3 percent. Consider walking or riding a bicycle instead of taking your usual cruise in the sedan.

Homes That Age Gracefully

As we live longer, our environmental needs often change. Perhaps we retire or start working from home; our children may move out or our parents may move in. We may decide to sell the big family house and move to a seaside condo, or closer to friends, theater, restaurants, museums, work, and other urban attractions. Perhaps we're looking for a home with fewer steps, wider doorways, guest rooms, or just more privacy. The "empty nest" may be just the excuse we need to spread our wings and explore a new environment or alter the one we have to maximize our space and our enjoyment of it.

Making sure that our home environment fits in with our changing needs throughout life is an important quality longevity goal. The trend today is toward openness and serenity in our living spaces, using fewer rooms and enjoying less clutter around us. If you have the means, simply tearing down walls to create larger spaces or adding walls to divide up separate rooms can often alter your home to meet your requirements.

If older parents are no longer able to live on their own, they may face the tough decision of either moving in with adult children, finding in-home care for themselves, selecting an assisted living facility, or choosing another option. If parent care becomes a reality for your family, consider the advantages and disadvantages of several housing choices:

- *Long-distance parent care.* Many parents prefer to live in their own, familiar home and neighborhood so they can continue getting the emotional and practical support of friends and community. This is offset, however, by the impractical drawback of family members living some distance away. Help with even minor tasks like a ride or simple errand may require searching for others to pitch in. A parent's illness or accident means the adult child may have to hop on a plane, which adds additional stress, cost, and inconvenience to family life.

- *Under the same roof.* If you have the room, an older parent may want to move in. Respecting each other's privacy while involving the parent in everyday family life helps with the transition. Live-in parents can often be helpful with babysitting or tutoring.

- *Assisted living and life-care communities.* Assisted living promotes the resident's independence while providing assistance with meals, support services, social activities, and twenty-four-hour supervision. Life-care communities offer different levels of care, ranging from independent housing to skilled nursing care. Many offer contracts guaranteeing lifetime shelter and care.

- *Nursing homes.* These provide the most intense level of care, including meals, skilled nursing, rehabilitation, medical services, personal care, and recreation. New, smaller homes with more domestic settings have a closer sense of community, and many traditional institutions are remodeling to create a more homelike environment. The AARP offers a checklist to help families choose a nursing home (*www.aarp.org/life/hous ingchoices/*).

An Ounce of Prevention

Facing new challenges and taking some risks can be exciting and adrenaline-boosting, while offering up new experiences and adventures. However, recklessness can shorten our life expectancy and should be avoided. Simple measures such as fastening seat belts, wearing helmets, and stowing or removing firearms from the house save lives every day.

As we go through the various stages of our lives, the challenges of keeping our environments safe will change. With young children in the house, the number one indoor danger is falling down stairs. Stairs can become an environmental danger for elderly people as well. Use of medications, visual impairments, and arthritis can also increase the risk of falling for older people. Ensuring proper lighting, avoiding clutter, and safely securing throw rugs are helpful preventive measures. Here are some additional suggestions for maintaining safety at home as we get older:

- *Install handrails.* These are relatively inexpensive alterations that can help people who are unsteady on their feet. Be sure to have at least one handrail on all stairways and steps, and ensure that they are securely attached.
- *Secure steps.* Check that stairs are in good shape and that they are slip resistant. Try adding a strip along the edge of each step in a contrasting color so it is easier to see, or use reflective antiskid treads.
- *Clear walkways.* Arrange to have leaves, snow, and ice removed on a regular basis. During winter months, be sure to use salt or sand to avoid ice accidents.
- *Grab bars in the bathroom.* Installing grab bars in the bathtub, shower, and by the toilet can help prevent household falls. In the tub, grab bars on a side wall and the back wall are helpful for getting in and out. For additional support in the shower, consider a bench for showering while seated.
- *Mats.* A rubber mat in the tub and a nonskid bath mat beside it will help prevent falls.

Conserving Our Environment

Many people are aware of the need to conserve our planet's rain forests, oceans, water supplies, wildlife, and other natural resources, especially as more countries move toward industrialization. Nearly 80 percent of Americans live in urban environments, where parks and green areas are welcome breaks from the pavement of our cities. In urban settings, these green public areas have been linked to extended longevity. Japanese scientists found an increased life expectancy of up to five years for older Tokyo citizens correlating to the space available for taking a stroll near their homes or apartments, as well as the proximity of parks and tree-lined streets.

Our ability to conserve energy, keep the environment green, recycle, and avoid wastefulness helps us feel good about ourselves, as well as our surroundings. Trees, plants, and flowers, whether they are indoors or outdoors, enhance our mental and physical well-being. Landscaping often becomes a focal point, adding texture and enlivening the environment.

Conservationists take advantage of natural cycles and use several waste products from one cycle to fuel another. Kitchen and bath water can be recycled into the yard, and kitchen and garden trimmings can be used as compost material. Edible landscaping is another option—a vegetable or herb garden is pleasing to the eye and can really come in handy when you need a sprig of rosemary or a few basil leaves to complete a culinary masterpiece.

Conserving resources and creating pleasant, clutter-free, and stress-free surroundings can help us achieve our quality longevity goals. Small changes in the way we design, build, and maintain our homes will save us money and energy, as well as increase our health and satisfaction. For example, technological advances have made it more efficient and less expensive to harness the sun's energy with solar paneling. Easy access to nontoxic house paint and natural wax and oils for floors and furniture can help keep our homes toxin-free. Installing low-flow faucets and dual-flush toilets helps conserve water. Buying appliances with a high-efficiency Energy Star rating by the Environmental Protection Agency (*www.energystar.gov*) can minimize energy consumption. And finally, in areas where rainwater is scarce, you might want to consider drought-tolerant landscaping using native plants.

Mastering Your Environment

- Bear in mind function and aesthetics when designing your home and work space. Try to control clutter and noise and arrange the bedroom in a way that enhances sleep and restfulness.
- Minimize your exposure to sun, smoke, mold, smog, and other airborne toxins.
- Stay safe on the road—let someone else drive if you can't handle it.
- Make your workplace safe and comfortable and consider ergonomic designs.
- Manage your technology to avoid information overload.
- If parent care becomes a reality, consider the advantages and disadvantages of various housing choices.
- Help conserve natural resources to protect your environment.

Essential 6

Body Fitness—Shape Up
to Stay Young

*My grandmother started walking five miles a day
when she was sixty. She's ninety-three today and we
don't know where the hell she is.*

— ELLEN DEGENERES

Alan F. was excited about his company's upcoming annual ski retreat. For the past few years, a knee injury and then a back sprain had kept him in the ski lodge Jacuzzi, while his wife enjoyed the slopes with assorted handsome young ski instructors. Months before this year's trip, Alan began a strengthening and flexibility program at his gym to make sure that his back was strong and his knee wouldn't give out. He also swam laps and did a stretching routine every morning. Alan gradually got stronger and more limber, and felt like his old self.

Alan was definitely psyched as he and his wife arrived at the ski lodge—this was *his* year to show the other guys at the conference that he could still ski the black diamond slopes. As his wife unpacked in their suite, he decided to run down to the fitness center to get on the treadmill before dinner. She heard the door shut as he left, but a couple minutes later she heard him come back in again. "That was a fast workout," she called to him. "Ice! I need ice!" he hollered from the other room as he limped to the sofa and elevated his leg. In his enthusiasm to get to the gym, he had skipped the elevator and instead raced down the stairs two at time. Missing a step, Alan had gone tumbling down the last three stairs. His right ankle was already starting to swell. By dinnertime, Alan had seen a doctor, who wrapped his badly sprained ankle, gave him a set of crutches, and banished his dreams of skiing for yet another year. Alan's wife offered to stay at the lodge and play chess with him the next day, but he wouldn't have it, insisting she take off for the slopes and perhaps get a lesson from one of the young instructors standing by. That night, when the other guys at the conference saw that Alan had already sprained his ankle, they figured he'd done it skiing—he didn't mention the treacherous, double-diamond stairway leading from his room to the gym.

Years ago, our ancestors didn't worry about getting enough exercise—they were too busy hunting and gathering to think about it. Today, our lifestyles tend to be more sedentary—we spend time sitting in front of computers, driving in cars, and watching our televisions, so many of us need to plan our daily physical exercise. Sticking with those fitness plans not only has a major impact on our health and youthfulness, but it also increases the number of years we can expect to live. Regular exercise adds quality to those extra years because it makes us feel better—physically and emotionally.

All forms of physical activity, whether it's walking, cycling, basketball, or dancing, appear to prolong healthy living. A study of more than sixteen thousand Harvard alumni, age thirty-five to seventy-four, found that regular physical activity can add at least a couple of years to life expectancy. They found that men who played tennis, swam, jogged, or took brisk walks had up to 33 percent lower death rates and a 41 percent lower risk of heart disease than their more sedentary colleagues. Studies of championship skiers and college athletes have found an increased lifespan of four or more years, as compared with the general population. Many sports and forms of exercise work both the mind *and* the body, and extend life as well as protect the brain.

We don't need to run a daily marathon to reap the benefits of exercise. Walking merely ten to fifteen minutes a day, or what adds up to approximately ninety minutes each week, significantly reduces the risk for developing Alzheimer's disease. Physically active people have lower rates of heart attacks, colon and breast cancer, diabetes, and depression, and these benefits accrue at almost any age. One study of more than four thousand volunteers found that physical fitness earlier in life was associated with better cardiac health later in life. Another recent study found that men taking up exercise, even after age sixty, can increase their life expectancy.

Becoming physically active on a routine basis may even boost your sex life. A study of approximately five hundred middle-aged men found that those who exercised regularly reported more frequent and satisfying sexual encounters than their less active counterparts. Another investigation found that the level of sexual activity of middle-aged expert swimmers was comparable to that of the average adult twenty years younger, *after* drying off.

Regular exercise fortifies muscles, tendons, and cartilage, and increases bone density—all important for keeping our bodies fit and young. The improved strength and balance we gain reduces the risk of falling and injury. Working out also gives us a sense of euphoria—sometimes referred to as a "runner's high"—by stimulating endorphins. Exercise boosts immune function, improves cardiac health, and increases circulation throughout the body. By helping to control body weight, exercise can lower the risk for diabetes, high blood pressure, and strokes.

Looking and Feeling Younger

Almost every magazine cover or television program reminds us that our culture emphasizes youth and beauty. And many people are motivated to remain physically active because it helps them look younger and more attractive. When someone makes a commitment to pursue a quality longevity program—eating the right foods, getting enough exercise and sleep, remaining involved and staying mentally active—they often shed pounds, feel an increase in strength and stamina, and appear younger and slimmer. They often start to get positive feedback from friends, family, and coworkers about how good they look, which leads to higher self-esteem, which further fuels their sense of youthfulness and attractiveness.

Youthful looks are often synonymous with beauty, and what we consider to be beautiful varies among cultures and has deep psychological roots. Historically, women have had much more pressure to appear young and attractive than men have had, although that is beginning to change. In Westernized societies, where there is little risk of seasonal lack of food, scientists have found that a woman's waist-to-hip ratio is a strong indicator of her attractiveness to men. This makes sense because waist size conveys information on her reproductive and health status.

Studies of self-perception of attractiveness find that women tend to select a relatively lean body image as the most desirable, attractive, and healthy one. Although this can be taken to the extreme in women who develop eating disorders, dissatisfaction with body size and a wish to be thinner generally motivates women to eat healthier diets. As a woman ages, she lets up a bit on what she sets as her ideal body weight. Systematic studies have found that over the age of thirty, a woman will rate her ideal figure as significantly larger than that perceived as most attractive to men.

When a person perceives beauty, it triggers a predetermined

physiological response in the brain. Dr. Itzhak Aharon and colleagues at the Harvard Medical School in Boston found that when a volunteer views a beautiful face, the brain activates a specific circuit involving the neurotransmitter dopamine. This is the same neural circuitry that controls eating, sexual appetite, making money, or seeking drugs. When dopamine is released in the brain, people experience a sense of pleasure that can be reinforced with repetition. This may explain why some people become obsessed with appearance and youthful looks in much the way that others become obsessed with food or addicted to drugs.

A sensible interest in maintaining an attractive appearance is a healthy and reasonable quality longevity goal. Feeling fit and attractive helps us to feel positive about ourselves and to remain socially connected. The Longevity Fitness Routine can improve our health and life expectancy, as well as provide the added benefit of making us look as good as we feel. Of course, many factors beyond physical appearance will influence our sense of attractiveness, including personality, accomplishments, self-confidence, mood, attitude, and external input. Many people have benefited from medical and surgical treatments in their pursuit of beauty and youthfulness (see Essential 8).

Pace Yourself

Baby boomers have come a long way from the physical education classes many recall from high school, when they had to run around a track, touch their toes, climb the ropes, and work out in ways that later in life might injure more than strengthen. Today we have numerous fitness regimens to choose from, and it is often best to sample several exercise techniques to discover what works best for each of us, paying particular attention not just to our health, but also to our enjoyment during workouts.

People with an ongoing medical condition should check with their doctor before starting any exercise program. Also, working out with a friend or in a group is a great way to get both physical *and* so-

Harry A., a seventy-year-old retired entrepreneur, was excited about his new workout routine. After a session with his trainer, he was determined to avoid the injuries he typically suffered whenever he took up an exercise program or sport. His tennis days were over after his amazing backhand tweaked his lower back. After three months of abdominal crunches and hamstring stretches, he was back on the golf course, until his upper back protested following an awesome 250-yard drive. Who would've thought that you needed to warm up before golf? His physical therapist recommended Pilates, which got him flexible enough to try the new elliptical machine his wife gave him for his seventieth birthday. The physical therapist had warned him to start out easy and build up his endurance gradually. Harry kept that advice in mind as he carefully mounted the elliptical machine, adjusted his heart-rate monitor strap, focused on his posture and breathing, and began to pedal. He pushed in all the right buttons and got the machine going at the right pace. As he pedaled, Harry kept murmuring to himself: "I will *not* overdo it . . . I will *pace* myself . . . I *will* stop when the timer goes off." He gradually increased his speed, kept his breathing steady, and he began to feel a little sweat break out. Whew boy, he was getting tired, but Harry kept pedaling, and then boom—he could feel that endorphin boost kick in! In fact, before he knew it, the timer-buzzer went off and he had finished his workout. Yes! He had made it through his first session with no injuries at all! He looked up at the timer—three minutes had elapsed. Tomorrow he would *really* go for it and bump the timer up to four minutes.

cial. You can increase your stamina through mutual encouragement while you chat about other things on your mind, which can reduce stress while it helps pass the time.

Although building up our exercise stamina gradually is best for avoiding injury, it is also important to push ourselves to the next level whenever we're ready, in order to gain the full benefits from our workouts. So-called weekend warriors—people who exercise only on weekends or once a week—may have a higher risk for injury and often don't get enough of a benefit from their exercise for it to be longevity-promoting.

Longevity Fitness Basics

To get our bodies in optimal shape so we can live healthier longer, our exercise routines should cover three fitness categories: *cardiovascular conditioning, balance/flexibility*, and *strength training*. Many exercises, including some of those described later in the Longevity Fitness Routine, provide benefits in more than one of these categories. When we do a series of strength-training exercises, we are also getting a certain degree of cardiovascular workout. Some exercise techniques, such as yoga or Pilates, have benefits in all three categories.

Depending on your goals and your baseline fitness level, you may want to emphasize one category more than the others, although all three are vital. If a person wants to lose weight, then increasing the duration and frequency of his or her cardiovascular conditioning workouts can help by burning more calories. Those with injuries might want to give extra focus to strength training, especially to the muscles around and supporting the injured area. Concentrating on balance and flexibility is crucial for everyone who wants to remain free of pain and avoid future injuries.

CARDIOVASCULAR CONDITIONING

Any continuous exercise we do to raise our heart rate will boost our cardiovascular fitness, and as more oxygen enters the bloodstream we get what is known as the aerobic effect. Regular cardiovascular workouts—running, cycling, aerobics, basketball, hiking, stair-stepping, rowing—will improve the efficiency of the heart, lungs, and circulatory system so that they can get more nutrients and oxygen to the muscles and other tissues. Such exercise routines also burn calories and help to keep weight down, lower blood pressure, strengthen immune system function, and reduce stress, as well as lower the risk for diabetes, dementia, and other age-related illnesses.

How much cardiovascular conditioning each person needs varies, depending on his or her age and general health. Although research generally shows greater cardiac benefit with longer exercise sessions, even brief but regular workouts are longevity-promoting. A recent study found that three ten-minute cardiovascular workout sessions—such as brisk walks—throughout the day provided as much benefit in lowering risk for heart disease as a single thirty-minute session.

We can get the most from our cardiovascular exercise by maintaining our target heart rate. To find this target rate, many experts suggest that the average person aim for somewhere between 70 and 90 percent of their maximum heart rate (see box).

Most fitness trainers recommend a warm-up phase before a cardiovascular workout, in order to increase body temperature and loosen joints. By also increasing the pulse rate slightly, it prepares the heart for a more vigorous workout. Warm-up phases usually include stretching and breathing exercises that may last from five to ten minutes. The actual workout phase can last anywhere from ten to sixty minutes, depending on your fitness level and your particular

Calculating Your Target Heart Rate

Your maximum heart rate can be calculated by subtracting your age from 220. A 50-year-old man would subtract 50 from 220, leaving 170—his maximum rate. Seventy percent of 170 is 119; and 90 percent of 170 is 153. So during his cardiovascular workout session, this man should aim for a heart rate of somewhere between 119 and 153.

Heart-rate meters, which are easily strapped around the chest and send moment-to-moment heart-rate information to a wristwatch receiver, are a convenient way to monitor your cardiovascular workouts as you build up to the higher end of your target heart rate. The information is also helpful in keeping you from surpassing your target rate and working harder than you need to in order to achieve optimal results.

goal, such as increasing cardiovascular health, building up endurance, or losing weight.

Longer and more frequent cardiovascular workouts burn more calories and make it easier to lose weight; however, it's best to build up gradually to avoid soreness and injuries. Also, try not to exercise right after a large meal, when a good deal of the body's blood supply goes to the stomach and intestines to help digestion, and blood flow to other organs is down. Whenever possible, look for opportunities throughout the day when you can add an extra pop of cardiovascular work, such as skipping the elevator and taking the stairs, or briskly walking to do a nearby errand instead of hopping in the car.

Each cardiovascular workout should be followed by a five- to ten-minute cool-down phase that helps to gradually bring the body's physiology back to its resting level, allowing the heart to adjust back to a slower, nonexercising rate of blood flow. Stretching your muscles after exercising will help avoid soreness and increase your flexibility.

Consider the following types of cardiovascular exercise, and choose one or more activities that you enjoy and that fit in with your lifestyle needs. Try varying your exercise options to keep your workouts interesting.

Walking. A brisk walk is an ideal cardiovascular activity for people at any age. Walking requires no training or special equipment, carries minimal risk of injury, and is one of the easiest exercise routines to fit into a busy schedule. You can increase the aerobic challenge of your walks by lengthening the duration or distance covered; or you may want to challenge yourself by walking up and down hills.

Jogging. Jogging provides more of a cardiovascular challenge than walking, and many joggers seem to be addicted to a "runner's high" from endorphin hormone boosts they often get during their workout. You can jog almost anywhere and in almost any climate, and it requires very little special gear, other than proper running shoes. Unfortunately, knee and back injuries force some joggers to switch to exercises that are gentler on the joints.

Swimming. This sport uses nearly all the major muscle groups, so it does an excellent job of getting our hearts pumping. Because it is a non-weight-bearing exercise, it is ideal for people who have suffered joint injuries from higher impact cardiovascular workouts.

Cycling. Another non-weight-bearing exercise, cycling, can be done outdoors, so you can enjoy the scenery or run an errand, or indoors on a stationary bike, while you read or watch TV. Spinning classes have become very popular and involve a class full of stationary bikers riding to upbeat music and the encouragement of an instructor. To maximize performance and avoid knee strain, make sure to adjust your seat height so that your leg is not quite fully extended at the bottom of the downward pedal.

Racquet Sports. Tennis and racquetball offer the thrill and satisfaction of a contest, as well as the challenge of improving your skills. For younger adults, injuries are relatively rare, but after years of wear and tear on their joints, some older adults choose to segue to lower-impact alternatives.

Dancing. Dancing not only offers a cardiovascular workout, it also improves balance and flexibility. Dancing has even been associated with a lower risk for developing Alzheimer's disease, perhaps because of the mental challenge one gets from learning and following new steps.

Aerobics Classes. Some people prefer working out in a group instead of going it alone, and aerobics classes are a fun way to get motivated through the encouragement of classmates and the instructor. Fast-paced aerobics classes provide a cardiovascular workout as well as training in motor skills and coordination. Many people alternate between aerobics classes and spinning classes (see above) to keep things lively.

Workout Equipment. Since most of us are not out getting our cardiovascular exercise working the fields, technology has caught up with our need for convenient and targeted workout equipment. Treadmills, stationary bicycles, rowing machines, and many other types of equipment make it easier to read or watch the news while getting in your daily cardiovascular exercise. One can also adjust the resistance and elevation of many machines in order to gradually build up endurance and avoid injury.

Step or stair-climbing machines not only burn calories efficiently, but they help give definition to the muscles of your lower body. However, because they tend to put stress on the knee joints, many people have moved on to the newer elliptical equipment, which glides the leg joints through an oval or elliptical movement. For people with knee problems, stationary bikes are another sensible alternative to treadmills or stair machines.

Housework and Gardening. Rhythmic tasks such as sweeping, mopping, raking, or hoeing provide an efficient cardiovascular workout, but if you don't do them routinely, be sure to warm up properly before working at too fast a pace, in order to avoid injuries. Basic chores can burn lots of calories—ten minutes of lawn mowing eats up about seventy-five calories; spend the same amount of time hedging and/or planting seeds, and you'll burn up about fifty calories. In addition to the health benefits, you get the chores done and save money by not hiring help.

BALANCE/FLEXIBILITY

Adding regular stretching and balance training to our fitness goals helps us maintain or regain better balance and coordination, and makes us less prone to injuries from falls. It also increases the flexibility of our muscles, which can improve our daily performance in everything—even tasks such as lifting, bending, or running to catch a bus. Stretching also helps keep our muscles from getting tight, which tends to improve posture and minimize aches and pains.

Balance is the body's ability to right itself. This capacity to remain stable on our feet involves *proprioception*, a mechanism that sends messages from the brain to the body and back, letting us know how to react and with how much tension in each muscle group. This system is generally automatic, but it can be enhanced through exercise and training.

Exercises to increase flexibility through stretching and other movements are key to the Longevity Fitness Routine. Not only does stretching reduce stress, decrease muscle soreness, and increase performance, it also helps us to relax during and after a workout. Although not all studies have confirmed that stretching exercises prevent injury, many do show benefits for specific muscle groups, such as the hamstrings behind the thighs, and the triceps muscles at the back of the arms. Traditionally, stretching is done as a warm-up to increase blood flow prior to a workout, and as a cool-down after a cardiovascular or strengthening session to increase flexibility while the muscles and tendons are still warm.

Stretching along with strengthening is important for maintaining *range of motion*, or the ability of a joint to bend and straighten. In healthy joints, movement increases blood flow, providing oxygen, nutrients, and lubrication to the joints, thus allowing smooth, pain-free movement. When joints move less, they become stiff and painful, which then discourages further movement. Balance and flexibility exercises encourage healthy movement, and help us to avoid pain and stiffness.

Although balance and flexibility exercises can involve fancy equipment, many of the best exercises require nothing more than a simple willingness to learn the movements. Just standing on one leg, walking heel-to-toe, or reaching your arms to the sky can be effective balancing and stretching exercises. The following are a variety of fitness approaches that improve balance and flexibility.

Tai Chi. This is an exercise that incorporates a series of slow and smooth movements that help reduce stress and promote relaxation (see Essential 4). Qi Gong is a related series of movements with less complicated stepping patterns. These movements are designed to stretch and lengthen muscles, ligaments, and tendons gently, increase breathing capacity, and loosen joints. They are especially helpful in improving balance and flexibility. A recent study found that tai chi exercises done three times a week for twelve weeks resulted in significant improvement in strength, mobility, and flexibility in older adults.

Yoga. Yoga's sequence of poses and breathing exercises not only helps us to relax (see Essential 4) but also improves balance and flexibility. The challenge of many yoga poses is to stay well aligned, which strengthens the muscles required for greatest stability.

Pilates. This exercise system focuses on flexibility, balance, and coordination, while increasing muscle strength and tone. Originally designed to help dancers recover from and avoid injuries, the exercises are performed in a specific order and require a small number of repetitions. The focus is on strengthening core muscles, which include the muscles of the stomach, lower back, buttocks, and inner thighs. Pilates also emphasizes control and form. Many exercises are basic enough to be done on a mat, while others require the assistance of an instructor and special Pilates machines. A basic mat program can be learned and performed at home with teaching aids such as videos or books.

Stability Balls. Also known as Swiss balls or exercise fitness balls, these items are becoming increasingly popular for home workouts, since they are relatively inexpensive and versatile. They introduce instability into any given exercise movement, which challenges us to work additional muscle groups beyond what the exercise was originally intended to work. Learning to do the exercises while balancing on the ball strengthens our muscles and increases our stability in everyday situations. Recent research found that stability balls are particularly effective in augmenting core strength and balance.

Balance Boards. These devices consist of boards atop cylinders or domes. Standing on the board and trying to maintain balance challenges our ability to remain stable. With practice, we can learn to do exercises on these boards, which can improve balance, coordination, strength, and range of motion. A recent study found that balance-board training significantly reduced the risk of ankle sprain, the most common sports injury.

STRENGTH TRAINING

Weight lifting and resistance training help increase the size and strength of muscles and fortify bones. Denser bones lower the risk for osteoporosis, making them less likely to fracture. Strength-building exercises also protect our joints, which can decrease pain from arthritis. These exercises also help stabilize blood sugar levels, which makes diabetes less likely. The lean body mass that forms as a result of strength training raises metabolic rates, which helps burn more calories throughout the day and can be helpful for weight control.

Strength training is not just for bodybuilders, athletes, or action heroes. In fact, older people seem to benefit the most from weight or resistance training. Studies have found that older men who spend three months doing weight training may be able to double or triple the strength and size of the large muscles in their upper legs. Even residents in nursing homes have shown dramatic improvements in strength and bone density from weight training.

Having well-balanced muscle groups will reduce the risk of injuries that occur when one muscle group is weaker than its opposing muscle group. The best way to avoid such muscular imbalances is to make sure that when you train a specific muscle group, you train the opposing muscle group, as well. For example, if you do several reps of biceps training for the muscle at the front of your arm, you would also want to work the opposing muscle, the triceps at the back of the arm, in order to remain balanced. It is also recommended that you start out by using a weight light enough to allow you to complete ten to fifteen repetitions of each exercise. As your strength increases, so should your weights.

Because strength training tears down muscle fiber, it is important to have adequate periods of rest between training sessions so muscles will repair and rebuild. We can do this by cross-training, or working out different muscle groups on alternate days, which allows for that kind of rest. You can train one group of muscles, such as your arms, shoulders, and chest on one day, and another group, your thighs, calves, and hamstrings, the following day. Many exercisers like to switch between cardiovascular workouts one day and strength-training sessions the next, while including a flexibility (stretching) and balance component in all their workouts. The following are some options to consider for your strength-training program.

Weight Machines. This equipment comes in many shapes and sizes and features pulleys that provide resistance throughout the weightlifting movement. Weight machines are relatively easy to use and can be safer than free weights because they guide the weightlifting motions and reinforce correct posture. Targeting specific muscle groups can often be easier to do with these machines than with free weights, because correct form must be learned and sustained for free weights to work effectively.

Free Weights. Because they allow us to work our muscles from any angle, free weights offer more versatility than weight machines, which have a limited number of functions. Free weights are also less expensive and are the fastest way to increase muscle strength and size. They help develop control, balance, and coordination. Proper instruction on correct form will increase the effectiveness of free-weight workouts and help people avoid injury.

Resistance Bands. Used for strength training as well as stretching exercises, these bands come in varying degrees of elasticity, and can be used to work out both upper and lower body muscle groups. As you build strength, you can wrap the band around your hands to make it tighter, increasing the resistance, or swap up to a higher-resistance band. Available at most drugstores or sporting-goods outlets, these lightweight resistance bands allow you to take your workout equipment with you wherever you go.

Pain-Free Fitness

As our bodies get older, injuries generally take longer to heal—we can't always just "walk it out" as we might have in our twenties or thirties. A minor back sprain or knee tweak may mean a week or two on ice before we bounce back to the racquetball court. But if we're not physically conditioned, flexible, and strong, we may not bounce back for much, much longer.

Approximately four out of five Americans suffer from intermittent or chronic back pain at some point during their lives. Fortunately, most back sufferers find relief and improvement through targeted exercise. The usual risk factors for low-back pain are weak abdominal muscles and limited flexibility.

Toning your stomach muscles with sit-ups, crunches, or other abdominal exercises helps to strengthen and protect your back and its surrounding muscles. By adding stretching exercises, your back and the muscles around it will become more flexible and elongated, protecting it from future injury and pain. The Pilates program is a great way to protect the back, with its focus on strengthening the "core" muscles—those around your trunk and pelvis—which support the spine and help to align the body correctly.

To work your body's core, engage your deepest abdominal muscle by coughing once. The muscle you feel contracting deep in your abdomen is your transversus abdominis. It isn't the only muscle that makes up your body's core, but by trying to keep this muscle contracted throughout the exercises, the rest of your core muscles get a workout, too.

In addition to the following Longevity Fitness Routine, which includes a series of stretching, strengthening, and toning exercises that protect the back, several other simple interventions can bring relief to back-pain sufferers. These include wearing low-heeled shoes; avoiding long periods of sitting by walking and stretching at regular intervals; bending your knees when lifting heavy objects; and sleeping on your side with a pillow between your knees. Overweight back sufferers may find that shedding a few pounds can help relieve some of the discomfort.

Many athletes and nonathletes alike suffer from knee problems, and this joint becomes more vulnerable with age. Strengthening the quadriceps muscles (front of the thigh), the inner and outer thigh muscles, and the smaller muscles and ligaments surrounding the kneecap can protect that area from injury and help keep the kneecap from sliding out of place. Several exercise-related knee problems can be easily corrected by wearing the proper footwear or shoe inserts. Running or power-walking on hard surfaces such as concrete may contribute to knee problems, and joggers tend to prefer softer dirt and gravel roads to run on. If you should experience knee pain while exercising, stop and apply ice as soon as possible. If the discomfort does not improve, consult your doctor.

Longevity Fitness Routine

You don't have to join a gym or buy any special clothing or high-tech equipment to begin an exercise routine that incorporates the three basic longevity fitness areas: cardiovascular conditioning, balance/flexibility, and strength training. All you need for your workout is a little time, a chair, and a bath towel. If you don't own any free weights you can start out by using sixteen-ounce soup cans instead, although once you build up your strength and endurance, you may wish to buy heavier dumbbells.

CARDIOVASCULAR CONDITIONING

If you are new to cardiovascular conditioning, try beginning with a brisk five-minute walk, then work up to ten minutes, then fifteen, and eventually twenty or more. It's a good idea to warm up before doing any type of sport or workout, and follow your cardiovascular or strengthening routine by stretching your muscles, to avoid soreness and increase flexibility. You can use some or all of the stretching exercises included in the Flexibility and Strengthening Workout below. You can do your cardiovascular conditioning on the same day as your strength training, or on alternate days, depending on your time and fitness level.

FLEXIBILITY AND STRENGTHENING WORKOUT

Begin this routine slowly, doing as many repetitions as you feel comfortable doing. Gradually, you will build up strength and stamina, and be able to increase your number of repetitions and sets, as well as the amount of weight you are lifting.

Alternating Overhead Stretch. This flexibility exercise helps improve range of motion in your arms, shoulders, and chest, as well as release muscle tension in your back and the sides of your trunk. Stand with your knees bent and feet hip-width apart. Raise both arms over your head and slowly reach for the ceiling, alternating your right and left arm. Keep your hips still and do twelve repetitions. Take a deep breath, and exhale as you bring your arms to your sides. Repeat the stretch two more times.

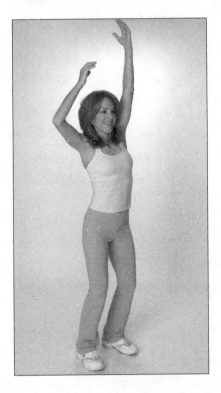

Alternating Overhead Stretch

Side Stretch. This stretch works the sides of the trunk and the waist. Stand with feet shoulder-width apart, and keep your knees slightly bent. Raise your right hand overhead and reach over to your left side as far as you can, then hold the position and breathe for a count of five. Slowly bring your torso upright while exhaling. Raise your left arm overhead, reaching to the right side as far as you can. Hold and breathe for a count of five. Slowly return to upright. Repeat both sides.

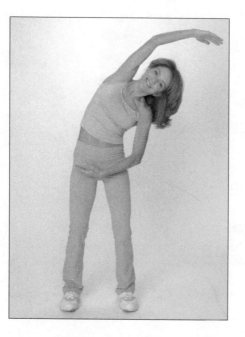

Side Stretch

Hip Stretch. The hip flexors help lift your leg in any position. Stretching the hip flexors helps to counter the prolonged hip flexion many of us experience by sitting for long periods of time. Stretching the muscles in front of your hips can help prevent "swayback" (a condition in which the spine is unnaturally arched backward).

Kneel on your left knee and extend your right leg in front of you, knee bent and foot flat on the floor. Shift your weight onto the bent right leg and press the right knee forward. Make sure the right knee does not extend past the right foot. Try to keep your pelvis tucked under and your abdominals pulled in. Feel the stretch through your left hip and thigh, as well as your right hamstring, as you breathe deeply for fifteen to thirty seconds. Relax, then repeat the stretch on the other side.

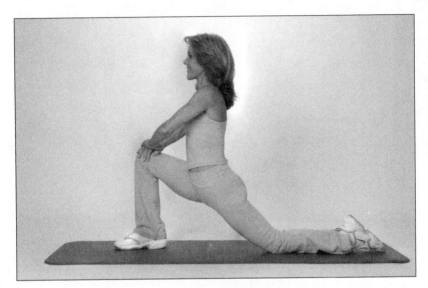

Hip Stretch

Quadriceps Stretch. Limber quadriceps muscles help us bend and straighten our legs, as well as lift and flex our knees. Steady yourself with your left hand on a chair back or wall, then bend your right leg behind you and grasp that ankle with your right hand. Keep your knees together and your standing leg slightly bent, as you gently pull your right foot closer toward your bottom. Feel the stretch through the front of your leg as you keep moving that foot back. Hold for a count of twelve and repeat on the other side. *Varia-*

tion: For extra balance work, try doing this stretch without holding onto anything.

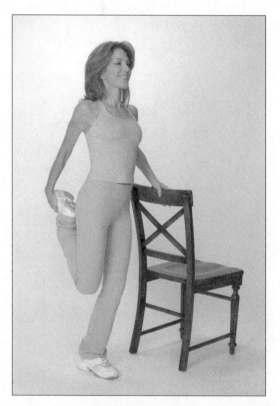

Quadriceps Stretch

Achilles Tendon Stretch. The Achilles tendon connects the leg muscles to the foot, allowing us to point our toes, rise on our toes, and walk. Correct stretching and warming up before a workout helps protect the Achilles tendon and its surrounding muscles.

Stand arm's length from a wall and place your hands flat against the wall in front of your shoulders. Lean forward and step your right leg straight back. Bend your forward knee and keep your right leg straight as you drop your right heel to the floor and push your chest forward. Feel the stretch through your right calf and hamstring muscles, as well as your Achilles tendon. Breathe and hold for a count of twelve, then repeat on the other side.

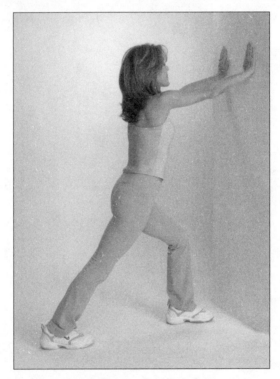

Achilles Tendon Stretch

Forward Leg Lifts. The next few exercises strengthen the muscles in the front, back, and side of the leg, protecting the knees, hips, and pelvis. Holding on to a chair back or wall with your left hand, slowly lift your right leg forward, keeping it straight with the toes pointed. Your standing leg should be slightly bent to protect your back from strain. Pause for a second with your leg in the up position and then slowly lower it. After ten repetitions, hold your right leg in the up position. Now bend your knee in, very slightly, and then straighten it, keeping the toes pointed. Do this ten times, then switch legs and repeat the series. *Variation: To work on your balance, try doing the exercises without holding on to anything.*

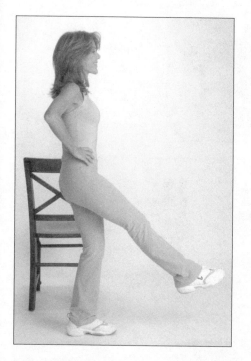

Forward Leg Lifts

Hip Abduction. Stand and hold on to a chair or wall with your left hand, keeping your left leg slightly bent, as you raise your *straight* right leg out to the side, foot flexed. Hold for a count of three, and then lower the leg. Do ten repetitions, keeping your hips and body straight during the exercise. Switch sides and repeat with the other leg. Work up to two sets.

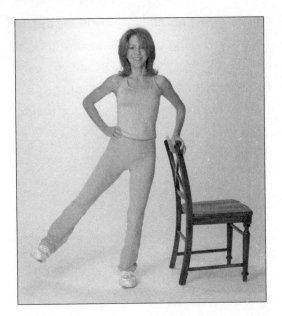

Hip Abduction

Hip Extension

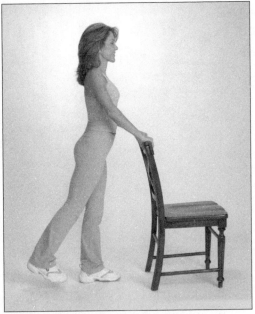

Hip Extension. Place both hands on the back of a chair. Hold your abdominal muscles tight and don't arch your back as you push your right leg straight behind you, until you feel a squeeze in the back of the thigh and buttocks area. Hold for a count of three, and release. Repeat ten times and then switch legs. *Variation: Try doing this exercise with the working leg bent at the knee, but after each push back, don't release the leg any farther forward than the standing leg.*

Chair Squat. This is a toner for the thighs, hips, and buttocks. Stand in front of a chair with your feet slightly more than hip-width apart, your toes pointed forward, and your arms crossed. Bend at your hips and lower your bottom to the chair. The moment you touch it, push up to standing. Repeat ten times. Gradually build up to twenty repetitions. *Variation: When you feel ready, try doing this exercise without the chair.*

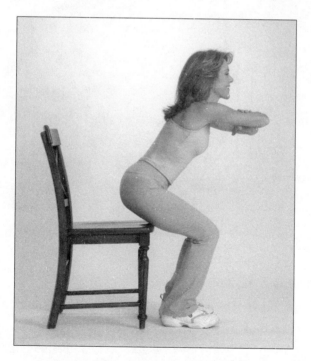

Chair Squat

Calf Strengthener. Stand on the balls of your feet on a first stair step. Raise your heels as high as you can, tightening your calf muscle. Pause for a moment, then slowly lower your heels until they're below the step and you feel a stretch in your calf muscle. Do ten repetitions. Build up to two to three sets.

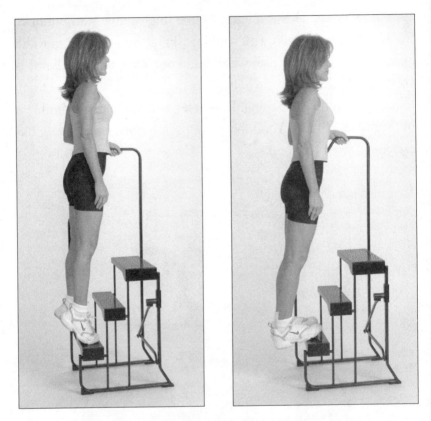

Calf Strengthener (Fig. A)   Calf Strengthener (Fig. B)

Biceps Curl. This exercise is a great way to strengthen the muscles in the front part of the upper arm. Stand upright with feet shoulder-width apart and knees slightly bent. Hold a set of dumbbells at your thighs, with your palms facing forward and your elbows anchored against your sides. Keep your back straight and abdominal muscles tight. Slowly raise both dumbbells toward your shoulders, making sure your elbows do not move, and do not rotate your wrists. Slowly lower to starting position, but don't fully extend your arms. Repeat twelve times. Gradually build up to three sets.

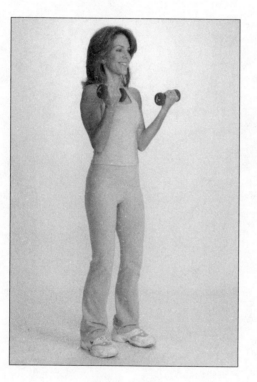

Biceps Curl

Upright Rows. The next two exercises benefit the upper back and shoulders. Stand with your feet shoulder-width apart and knees slightly bent. Hold a dumbbell in each hand in front of your thighs, palms facing in. Inhale as you raise both dumbbells up to just under your chin, with your elbows bent at shoulder height. Hold there a moment and then slowly exhale as you lower your arms to the starting position. Keep the dumbbells close in to your body throughout the exercise. Repeat ten to twelve times and gradually build up to two sets.

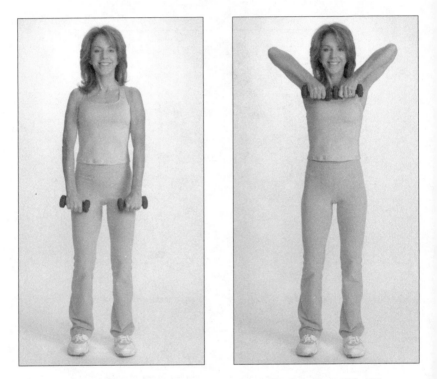

Upright Rows (Fig. A)   Upright Rows (Fig. B)

Lateral Lift. Stand upright with feet shoulder-width apart and knees slightly bent. Hold the dumbbells at your sides, with your palms facing each other. Raise both arms to the sides until they're shoulder height, and keep your elbows slightly bent. Pause for a moment and then slowly return to the beginning position. Repeat twelve times. Build up to three sets.

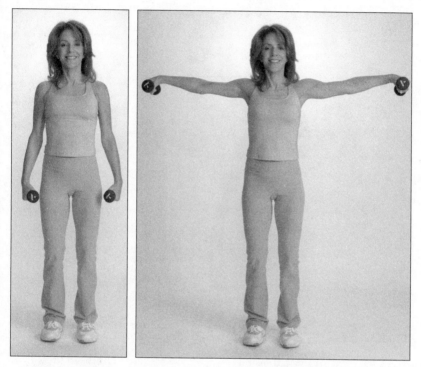

Lateral Lift (Fig. A)   Lateral Lift (Fig. B)

Triceps Extension. This will strengthen and tone the muscles in the back of the upper arm. Hold a dumbbell in your right hand and place your left hand on a chair back. With your feet shoulder-width apart and knees bent, keep your back straight and lean forward, bringing your right elbow back to shoulder height with the arm bent at a right angle. Slowly extend your arm from the elbow until the arm is straight and the head of the dumbbell is pointing up. Hold a moment and slowly return the weight to the starting position, keeping the upper arm and elbow still. Do ten to twelve repetitions on each arm. Build up to two sets.

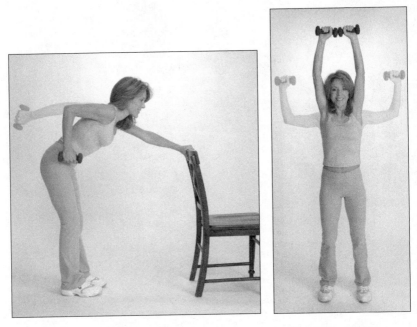

Triceps Extension   Overhead Press

Overhead Press. This works the shoulders, the triceps, and the upper back, and helps develop overhead lifting strength. Stand upright with feet shoulder-width apart and knees slightly bent. Hold a dumbbell in each hand, out to your sides at shoulder height. Bend your arms to ninety-degree angles, with your palms facing forward. Be sure to keep your back straight and your head in line with your spine as you press the weights together straight up over your head, without locking your elbows. Hold a moment, then return to the starting position. Repeat ten times. Work up to two sets.

Shoulder Stretch. You have worked your upper and lower body, so it is time for some more stretches. Reach one straight arm across your chest toward the other shoulder. With the opposite hand, grasp your elbow and pull your arm in as close to your body as possible. Hold for a count of ten, then release and stretch the other side for a count of ten.

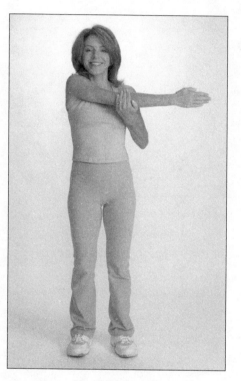

Shoulder Stretch

Upper Arm Stretch. Raise both arms overhead. Bend the right elbow, dropping the right hand behind your head. Hold the bent right elbow with your left hand and pull it down and back behind your head. Feel the stretch in your right triceps muscle and shoulder. Hold for a count of ten, and then repeat on other side.

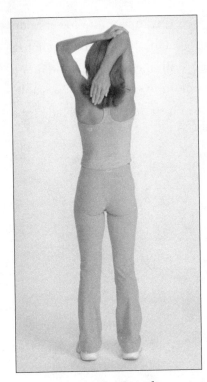

Upper Arm Stretch

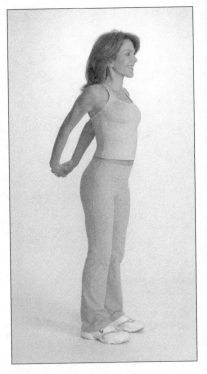

Chest Stretch

Chest Stretch. Clasp your hands behind your back. While keeping your chest high, lift your arms straight up behind you. Hold the stretch for fifteen seconds, then repeat. For a greater challenge, bend forward and raise your arms up higher.

Cat Stretch. This is a yoga movement designed to relax the lower back and pelvic area. It can also help release tension in the shoulders and upper back. On hands and knees, exhale as you pull your belly in, drop your head, and arch your back up toward the ceiling as high as possible—like a cat stretching. Hold for a count of two. Now slowly inhale, raising your head to look upward, and lowering your back into a scooped or bowl position for the opposite stretch. Repeat four to five times, keeping the motions fluid.

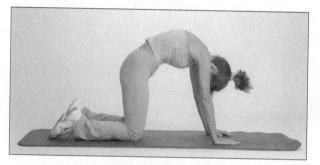

Cat Stretch (Fig. A)

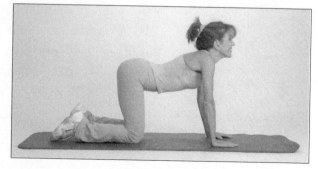

Cat Stretch (Fig. B)

Hamstring Stretch. Hamstring muscles in the back of the thigh work in opposition to the quadriceps in the front; however, they lag behind in strength and flexibility. Without proper stretching, they may be prone to injury and "pulls" from sudden movements. Lie on your back with your legs extended. Bring in one knee and wrap a towel around the arch of that foot. Holding the towel with both hands, gently straighten that leg toward the ceiling as much as possible. Use the towel to keep pulling the leg toward your nose. Hold for three to five deep breaths, then switch legs.

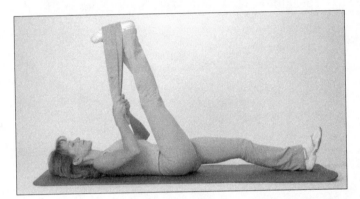

Hamstring Stretch

Abdominal Crunch. No strengthening routine is complete without working the abdominals, or core. Lie on your back with your knees bent, feet flat on the floor. Lace your fingers behind your head, keeping your elbows pointed out. Take a deep breath. As you

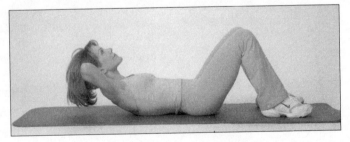

Abdominal Crunch

exhale, pulling your navel down toward your spine, raise your upper torso off the floor and push your lower back into the floor. Focus on using your lower abdominal muscles without straining your neck. Hold for a moment and then release slowly. Complete a set of ten, but as soon as you are able, build up to five or more sets.

Abdominal Side Toning. This exercise for toning the lateral abdominal muscles is sometimes called the "bicycle." Lie on your back with hands clasped behind your head. Raise your knees directly above your hips with calves parallel to the ground. Take a deep breath. As you exhale, lift your head, torso, and *left* elbow toward your *right* knee, while pushing your *left* leg out straight. Hold for one count, then switch to the other side, lifting your head, torso, and *right* elbow toward your *left* knee, and pushing your *right* leg out straight. Be sure to pull your navel in toward your spine with each exhale and contraction. Do a set of ten repetitions on each side, increasing the number of sets over time.

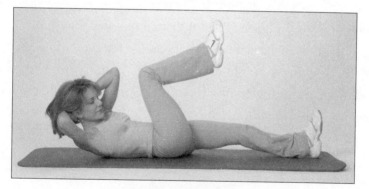

Abdominal Side Toning

Pelvic Tilt. This exercise strengthens the muscles in your buttocks, hamstrings, and abdominals, while it gently stretches the lower back. Lie on your back with your knees bent and feet shoulder-width apart on the floor. First, tighten your stomach mus-

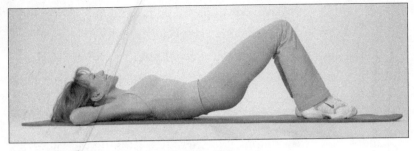

Pelvic Tilt

cles, then raise your buttocks off the floor slightly, tightening them. Be sure to keep your middle-to-lower back on the floor. Hold for a moment, then release. Repeat twelve to twenty times. *Variation: To notch it up a bit, raise your buttocks up about six inches from the floor while keeping your stomach and buttocks tight. Hold for a count of three and repeat twelve times.*

Back Leg Lift. Lie on your stomach with your legs straight and your hands folded under your cheek or chin. Tighten your stomach muscles, then lift your right leg two to three inches off the floor, tightening your buttocks. Hold it there a moment and lower it, and repeat the movement with your left leg. Do ten repetitions on each side. By keeping your stomach and your buttocks muscles tightened, and not lifting too high, you will protect your lower back. *Variation: Bend the lifting leg.*

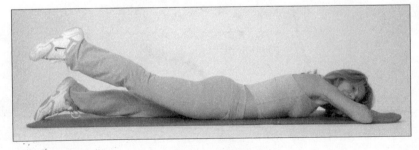

Back Leg Lift

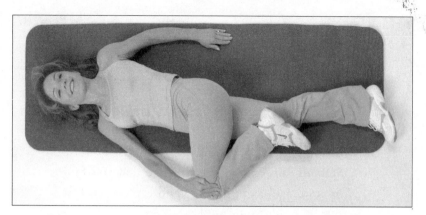

Hip Twist

Hip Twist. Lie on your back with your legs extended straight out on the floor. Slowly bend your left knee and bring it across your body to the right, until you feel a stretch in the lower back and hip area. Hold for a count of twelve. Return to starting position and repeat with the other leg.

Upper-Body Floor Stretch. Lie on your stomach with your palms on the floor, under your shoulders. Keeping your pelvis and thighs on the floor, slowly push your shoulders up until your arms are as straight as possible. Feel the stretch through your chest, shoulders,

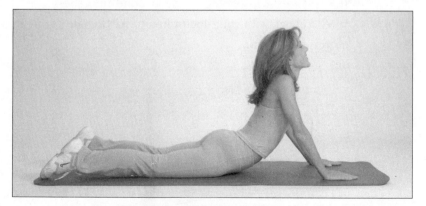

Upper-Body Floor Stretch

and back. Hold for a count of five, and then lower to the floor. Repeat two or three times.

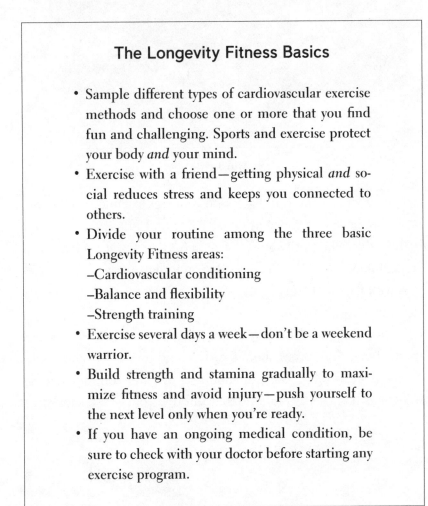

The Longevity Fitness Basics

• Sample different types of cardiovascular exercise methods and choose one or more that you find fun and challenging. Sports and exercise protect your body *and* your mind.

• Exercise with a friend—getting physical *and* social reduces stress and keeps you connected to others.

• Divide your routine among the three basic Longevity Fitness areas:
  –Cardiovascular conditioning
  –Balance and flexibility
  –Strength training

• Exercise several days a week—don't be a weekend warrior.

• Build strength and stamina gradually to maximize fitness and avoid injury—push yourself to the next level only when you're ready.

• If you have an ongoing medical condition, be sure to check with your doctor before starting any exercise program.

Essential 7

The Longevity Diet

All you need is love. But a little chocolate now and then doesn't hurt.

— CHARLES M. SCHULZ

You're halfway through a long business trip, exhausted after visiting five cities in three days. You almost missed your last connection and couldn't grab anything to eat at the airport. It's midnight when you finally check into your hotel room, too tired to even call room service. Hell, maybe skipping a meal will help you lose those six pounds that have crept on. You get ready for bed and scan the room for some bottled water, when you spot it—the *minibar*. You steel yourself and head toward it with determination: You're just getting a cold bottle of water and you're out of there—no chips, no cookies, and absolutely, for *damn* sure, you are *no way* checking out the candy shelf. Right—there's peanut M&M's, chocolate-covered mints, a KitKat bar, and a giant Snickers. The Snickers only has 170 calories per serving . . . *That's* not bad . . . You fold back the wrapper—just enough to have a couple of bites, as you flip on the TV. The entire bar is long gone before you glance around and realize you never got that water . . .

For as much time as we spend thinking, talking, and reading about food, many people still make the wrong choices about what they eat. Despite the greater attention placed on diets today, for health and weight loss, many still wonder *how much* to eat and *which* foods are healthy. Lots of people continue to ask the basic question: Can food that tastes good still be good for me? The answer is yes.

What we eat directly impacts our health and life expectancy by affecting our risk for heart disease, cancer, and other age-related illnesses. A large-scale, ten-year study found that people living a healthy lifestyle and eating a diet rich in antioxidant fruits and vegetables, olive oil and other monosaturated fats, as well as poultry and fish, had a 50 percent greater likelihood of living longer than study volunteers eating a less healthy diet.

Food also greatly affects our appearance and mental state. People often feel better about themselves when they look healthy and trim, and this has kept millions of people on various diets for decades—going up and down on the scale and wreaking havoc on their bodies. One of the biggest problems with many of today's popular diets is that they are hard to stick with for more than a few weeks or months, so people seldom get to enjoy the long-term health benefits. They tend to gain back all the weight they lost— and more. Often these diets fail because they leave people feeling not just bored, but deprived—whether it's a craving for carbohydrates, an urge to supplement calories to ease hunger pangs, or a desire to break down and splurge on a slice of chocolate cake or other favorite food.

Enter the Longevity Diet, which allows you to enjoy the foods you love (including that chocolate cake on occasion), trains you to add a variety of delicious and healthy foods, and emphasizes mindful awareness, so you know when you have had enough. Just as fitness experts put emphasis on cross-training our bodies—combining different forms of exercise in consecutive workout sessions in order to maximize results and minimize boredom—the Longevity

Diet teaches us to cross-train our meals, allowing us to break free of the repetition and boredom of many of today's popular food plans.

Cross-Train Your Diet for Longevity

Every day you will enjoy foods from the three major food groups that are scientifically associated with longer, healthier living:

- *Antioxidant fruits and vegetables* — Rich in vitamins, minerals, and phytonutrients, they taste great, fight disease, and add endless variety to our menus.
- *Proteins, lean meats, and healthy fats* — Supplying essential amino acids that maintain and repair the body's cells, they satisfy hunger the longest. Ocean-caught (wild) fish and nuts are particularly good sources of omega-3 fats, which protect not only the heart, but the brain, as well.
- *Whole grains, legumes, and other carbohydrates* — Packed with fiber and cancer-fighting nutrients, these carbohydrates provide immediate energy and keep the digestive system on track.

The *cross-training* component helps your body maintain a balance of these three food groups, and keeps your diet interesting and appealing by shifting the emphasis among the groups throughout the day. Using your imagination, think of meals as major motion pictures *starring* one of the three food groups. No single food group can star in all three movies (meals) in any given day. If you are trying to lose weight, protein — with its ability to provide essential nutrients and satisfy hunger the longest — should *star* in two of your meals each day.

If a fresh grilled salmon steak is the *star* of tonight's dinner performance, then steamed broccoli, wild rice, and a dinner salad with olive oil vinaigrette dressing might all play minor roles. And, of course, there is always a healthy dessert after dinner. Earlier in the day, you cross-trained your other meals as well: Perhaps oatmeal gave whole grains the starring role at breakfast, backed up by skim milk (protein) and sliced melon as supporting characters. Lunch showcased a crispy Chinese chicken salad, filled with colorful vegetables and orange slices in starring roles, with a small portion of chicken and sesame oil dressing playing bit parts.

Integral to the Longevity Diet are the midmorning and midafternoon snacks. Besides providing the energy we need to carry us between meals, these snacks ensure that our blood sugar remains steady throughout the day, which not only keeps us from feeling hungry but lowers our risk of developing diabetes and other diseases. We integrate cross-training into our snacks by combining the quick and tasty energy boost we get from carbohydrate-containing whole grains, fruits, or crunchy vegetables together with the sustained gratification of an ounce or two of protein, such as yogurt, string cheese, or perhaps a handful of almonds.

For those of us (hello!) who like a little nibble at night while reading or watching a movie, the diet also includes the option of having a third snack later in the evening—or, you can always save your after-dinner dessert to enjoy as your *nighttime snack*. For a more restful sleep as well as for weight management, try to limit these later snacks to something light and healthful. Good choices include fresh fruit, frozen fruit-juice bars, fresh or frozen yogurt, air-popped popcorn, and many other delicious and healthy alternatives.

The Longevity Diet not only promotes longer life but lets us toast to it with a glass of wine or other alcoholic beverage each day. Scientific evidence shows that drinking in moderation may protect the heart, lower risk for diabetes, and boost immunity and brain fitness. Scientists have found that on average, people who drink a glass of wine every day have less body fat and narrower waistlines than heavier drinkers or people who don't drink at all. Other research has shown that a daily glass of wine may help protect us against developing ulcers, gastritis, and stomach cancers.

So, you may be wondering, when do we get to eat the chocolate cake? Is now too soon? Cake is usually pretty loaded with sugar and fat, but at the end of a cross-training diet day, perhaps one that has been somewhat low in carbohydrates and fats, an occasional portion-conscious serving of cake at dessert time is fine. Tomorrow, go back to mixed berries or a scoop of sorbet for dessert. It's all good, and you won't feel deprived—you've stayed on your diet and you have nothing to feel guilty about. You've had your cake and eaten it, too!

Because the diet is designed to last for the long haul, it includes the food category I call *cheat eats*. These are any foods you love, crave, have to have and can't believe could be allowed on *any* diet, anywhere. For some, it's key lime pie; others may pine for a delicate foie gras; or perhaps it's deep-dish pizza with three cheeses that rings your bell. Okay, so those are my top three cheat eats—and I have been able to routinely work them into my program just fine. Including cheat eats in your diet has a scientific rationale: Evidence linking healthy diet choices to longevity has shown that you can include an occasional treat.

If your goal is to lose weight, you should consider putting cheat eats on hold, and increasing your exercise program—the old adage of "more calories out than in" still holds when it comes to shedding pounds. After an initial weight-loss period, a portion-controlled amount of your favorite cheat eat is a reasonable Saturday night dividend for a week well invested in the Longevity Diet. Later, we'll learn how to adjust the diet to lose weight quickly.

It is vitally important to remain hydrated throughout the day by drinking at least eight glasses of water. Not only will this help minimize hunger between meals and snacks, but it has been scientifically shown to increase metabolism, allowing our bodies to burn calories more quickly. A recent study found that after volunteers drank seventeen ounces of water, their metabolic rates increased by 30 percent, and the increases lasted nearly an hour. Try starting each new day by drinking a cool glass of water. It refreshes and cleanses the body, while helping to relieve any dehydration effects that may have occurred while sleeping.

Avoiding excess salt in our food helps us control our blood pressure, which lowers the risk for strokes, heart attacks, and kidney disease. Besides weaning ourselves off the salt shaker, we need to keep an eye on canned and frozen foods, prepared meals, and fast food, which usually has high salt levels.

A key to the success of the Longevity Diet is developing mindful awareness of how our bodies feel before, during, and after eating. Although dining can be one of life's greatest pleasures, many people living today's high-pressure, multitasking lifestyle have allowed eating to become little more than a habit, and certainly less satisfying than it could be. Some people tend to eat mindlessly while working, watching TV, talking on the phone, or during any number of other distractions or activities. Although meal time is a great opportunity to converse with family and friends, it is still vitally important to focus attention on:

1. How hungry we actually are before we begin eating, in order to gauge what portion size we really should take.
2. The moment-to-moment taste experience we have while eating, which allows us to slow down and savor our meals.
3. The increasing sense of fullness in our stomachs as we dine, and an awareness of when we are sated and have had enough.

Mindful eating not only helps us maintain an awareness of when we have had enough food, but also when we have had enough of a specific taste. Usually, after four or five bites of a particular food, taste buds become desensitized to that food's flavor. That is why even if someone cannot possibly eat another bite of grilled chicken, they may still have room for chocolate soufflé. Developing an awareness of this taste-specific satiety can help control binging and steer people away from unwanted calories.

Training yourself to use this and other mindful awareness eating techniques will not only help you *enjoy* meals more, you will most likely eat less and make healthier choices. You may notice the unique flavor of lemon juice on certain fresh vegetables, or a particular olive-oil vinaigrette dressing that you didn't realize you liked so much—both of which will help you eat more nutritiously. As you become more aware of how you feel before, during, and after eating—full, tired, energized, bloated—portion control will become easier, because you will have learned just how much food your body needs to feel good, as well as what foods make you feel energized and healthy. Also, stopping eating at the first sign of satiety is a great way to lose unwanted pounds without even trying, as well as maintain your target weight.

The Healthy Longevity Food Groups

To begin the Longevity Diet, familiarize yourself with the three major quality longevity food groups and the many food choices available in each of them. Each group has a list that includes several food suggestions, some of which you may already enjoy often, and some of which you may be less familiar with. Experimenting with various foods from the lists is a great way to expand your palate and increase your menu repertoire. I also encourage you to add other favorite healthy foods to your lists to help personalize your diet and keep it working for you for years to come.

ANTIOXIDANT FRUITS AND VEGETABLES

Just as metal gets rusty from being exposed to moist air, our bodies are vulnerable to oxidants, known as *free radicals*. We can't avoid free radicals, because they're everywhere—in our food, water, and air, and they also come from within us, as the by-products of our own metabolism. Many experts believe free radicals are the true culprits of aging. Our bodies are constantly under attack by free radicals and these attacks, collectively called oxidative stress, promote aging and diseases such as cancer, cataracts, arthritis, Alzheimer's, and heart disease.

We *can* fight back against free radicals by eating foods containing antioxidants such as vitamins A, E, and C; beans, broccoli, and dark leafy greens, such as spinach; and colorful fruits, such as blueberries, strawberries, and apples. Eating tomatoes, which contain the potent antioxidant lycopene, may also lower the risk for prostate cancer. We can get additional antioxidant vitamins by taking supplements (see Essential 8). I also recommend taking a multivitamin as well as a 500 mg (milligram) vitamin C tablet daily.

The box on page 191 contains a list of some healthy antioxidant fruits and vegetables, which will help you plan your Longevity Diet meals and snacks.

PROTEINS, LEAN MEATS, AND HEALTHY FATS

This food group gives us long-lasting appetite satisfaction while helping us to achieve and maintain our ideal body weight. Healthy proteins and fats also help us avoid age-related illnesses such as Alzheimer's and heart disease. Proteins, made up of amino acids, are the major structural component of all the body's cells and the enzymes that keep those cells functioning. Of the twenty vital amino acids our bodies need to function, nine of them—the *essential*

Antioxidant Fruits and Vegetables

Fruits	Mangos	Carrots
Apricots	Melons:	Cauliflower
Avocados	cantaloupe,	Celery
Berries:	honeydew	Corn
blackberries,	Nectarines	Cucumbers
blueberries,	Papayas	Eggplant
cranberries,	Peaches	Garlic
raspberries,	Pears	Green, leafy
strawberries	Pineapples	vegetables:
Cherries	Plums	cabbage, lettuce,
Citrus: grapefruit,	Tomatoes: Tomato	spinach, Swiss
oranges,	juice, V-8,	chard
tangerines,	tomato sauce	Juices: from any
tangelos, lemons,		vegetable
limes	**Vegetables**	Kale
Dried fruits:	Alfalfa sprouts	Mushrooms
apricots, prunes,	Asparagus	Onions
raisins	Beets	Winter squash
Frozen juice bars	Bell peppers	Zucchinis
Grapes	Broccoli florets	
Kiwi	Brussels sprouts	

amino acids—cannot be synthesized by our bodies and must be gotten through our diet.

Animal proteins such as fish, poultry, meat, eggs, milk, yogurt, and cheese supply these nine essential amino acids, and are therefore considered *complete* proteins. Plant proteins such as nuts, seeds, legumes, and grains are often called *incomplete* proteins because they can be deficient in one or more of the essential amino acids. Soybeans, a type of legume, are unique because they contain all of the amino acids needed to make a complete protein, just like meat. They also contain isoflavones, a plant-based compound that may reduce the risk of some types of cancer. Many foods are made from soybeans, including tofu. Another way to get soy into our diet is through soy protein isolate powder, which can be mixed into a smoothie with fruit, or stirred into oatmeal. People on vegan diets can get adequate complete proteins by combining their sources of incomplete proteins, making sure they get all of the essential amino acids each day.

Milk and other dairy products are high in calcium and not only strengthen bones but also lower the risk of developing colon cancer. A recent analysis of ten large studies found that people who drank more than one eight-ounce glass of milk each day were significantly less likely to develop colon cancer than those who drank less than two glasses per week. Other studies suggest that increased calcium, particularly from lowfat and nonfat dairy foods, may not only help people lose weight, but may assist baby boomers in controlling the expanding waistlines that sometimes accompany middle age.

Many protein-rich foods contain fat, which is often mistakenly regarded as a dietary taboo—just check out the numerous food labels highlighting fat-free this or lowfat that on the container. Many people don't realize that there are some health benefits to eating a certain amount of fat, as long as it's the *right type* of fat. Scientific evidence has shown that foods high in omega-3 fats, such as fish, olive oil, and soy products, reduce the risk for cardiovascular disease, stroke, and Alzheimer's disease.

A study recently published in the journal *Nature* found that olive oil contains a natural form of the common anti-inflammatory drug ibuprofen (marketed as Advil or Motrin), which could explain why eating olive oil may lower the risk of cancer, heart disease, and Alzheimer's disease. Our UCLA research team has found that ibuprofen and another common anti-inflammatory drug, naproxen sodium (marketed as Aleve), have the ability to actually dissolve the abnormal protein plaques that are thought to cause Alzheimer's disease.

We want to avoid foods high in saturated fats, trans fats, and omega-6 fats, including many cuts of beef, poultry fat, butter, cream, whole milk, tropical oils (e.g., palm, coconut), and many frozen and canned foods (check the labeling for contents). Trans fats are often found in commercially baked goods (e.g., packaged cookies, cakes, and crackers), which also tend to contain high amounts of white sugar and flour. These unhealthy fats are known to raise "bad" LDL cholesterol levels, which increase the risk for heart disease and other ailments.

Eating foods containing small amounts of healthy fats helps our bodies absorb essential vitamins and protects our cell membranes. It also helps to satisfy our hunger so we consume fewer calories overall. It is recommended that we limit added fat to no more than six teaspoons for an average two-thousand-calorie day. However, if you are a small or inactive person, you will burn fewer calories each day and should consider consuming less fat and fewer calories. A recent study found that restaurant diners who dipped their bread in olive oil (omega-3) actually ate less total bread and took in fewer calories than diners who used butter (omega-6). I'm not encouraging the consumption of mass quantities of bread and oil; but a limited amount of olive or walnut oil for a salad or a bit of sesame oil in a stir-fry makes a tasty and healthy addition to a meal.

The American Heart Association recommends eating fish twice a week in order to get enough omega-3 fats. Fish-eaters tend to have lower rates of arthritis and may have a lower risk for depression and some cancers. Wild salmon, halibut, light tuna, cod, flounder, sole, sea bass, shrimp, lobster, scallops, and crab are excellent choices. Farmed fish should be avoided, since it has more total fat than wild, and the additional fat is largely omega-6. But eating too much fish may lead to increased body levels of mercury, which can cause fatigue, hair loss, and other symptoms. Larger fish such as shark and swordfish tend to have higher mercury levels per ounce than smaller fish such as salmon or sole, which may be wiser choices.

Use the following list of proteins, lean meats, and healthy fats to help plan your meals and snacks.

Proteins, Lean Meats, and Healthy Fats

Beef (lean cuts)
Chicken breast
Cheese—nonfat or lowfat
  cottage, cream (light),
  goat, mozzarella, ricotta,
  Swiss
Eggs (egg whites preferred)
Fish: anchovy, bluefish,
  halibut, herring, mackerel,
  salmon, sardines, sea bass,
  trout, tuna, whitefish
Milk: lowfat or nonfat (skim),
  soy milk (lowfat)

Nuts: walnuts, peanuts
  (actually a legume),
  almonds
Peanut butter
Seeds and oils: canola,
  flaxseed, olive, sesame,
  sunflower, walnut
Soy proteins: soy protein
  isolate powder, soy meat
  substitutes, soy cereals, tofu
Turkey breast
Yogurt: high-quality lowfat or
  nonfat

WHOLE GRAINS, LEGUMES, AND OTHER CARBOHYDRATES

Studies have found that whole-grain and high-fiber foods help control weight gain, lower blood pressure, prevent strokes, and reduce the risk for diabetes and heart disease. Carbohydrates are the body's main source of energy, and this food group's multitude of choices are some of the most delicious and satisfying foods on the Longevity Diet. Steaming brown-rice risotto with seafood, a crust of fresh whole-grain bread, and a crisp vegetable salad is a meal that sounds good to me on any diet.

Whole grains, unlike many processed ones, contain vitamins, fiber, minerals, phytochemicals, plant proteins, and other healthful ingredients. They are absorbed by the body much more slowly then processed foods are. Whole-wheat bread, brown or wild rice, oatmeal, whole-grain pasta, and even popcorn are common sources of whole grains.

The fiber component of whole-grain carbohydrates cannot be

The Glycemic Index System

All carbohydrates are made up of sugar molecules. After we eat and digest them, these sugars, known as glucose, end up in our blood system. A method for classifying carbohydrates in which 0 refers to the healthiest carbohydrate and 100 the unhealthiest is known as the glycemic index, or GI. The GI measures how fast and how far blood sugar rises after we eat a food that contains carbohydrates. The carbohydrate's underlying structure is what influences its GI rating and determines how easily it can be digested. "Instant" foods are digested and absorbed into the bloodstream very quickly and thus have a high GI rating, much like a piece of white bread, which has a high GI score, and causes blood sugar to spike rapidly when eaten. Munch on some brown rice (low GI rating), on the other hand, and you'll digest more slowly, causing a lower and gentler change in blood sugar. Also, carbohydrate foods with added fat or acid (vinegar, lemon juice) are absorbed into the bloodstream more gradually. High-GI diets are not considered longevity-promoting, since they increase the risk for diabetes and heart disease. The table on pages 196–197 gives examples of GI ratings for common foods.

broken down by the digestive system, so it moves through and keeps everything moving along with it in a healthful way. This is partially why eating fiber-rich whole grains and other high-fiber foods protect against constipation, hemorrhoids, and diverticulosis. High-fiber whole grains also lower our risk for cancer of the colon, rectum, stomach, pancreas, endometrium, ovary, and prostate. When food manufacturers process carbohydrate products, they remove much of the fiber, which increases the food's glycemic index (see box). Processing also removes many vitamins, minerals, and phyto-nutrients.

An easy way to get whole grains into your diet is to add them to recipes you already make without whole grains. Try adding wild

How Much Common Foods Spike Blood Sugar

Minimal (Glycemic Index < 40)

Apples	Lima beans
Apricots, dried	Nonfat yogurt
Cherries	Peanuts
Fettuccine	Skim milk
Lentils	Soybeans

Low (Glycemic Index 40–54)

Baked beans	Oranges
Bran cereal	Orange juice
Canned chickpeas	Oatmeal
Cooked carrots	Spaghetti
Grapes	Unsweetened apple juice

Moderate (Glycemic Index 55–70)

Bananas	Oat-bran cereal
Brown rice	Pineapples
Natural muesli cereal	Whole wheat bread

High (Glycemic Index 71–84)

Bagels	Jelly beans
Cocoa Puffs	Pretzels
Cheerios	Puffed-wheat cereal
Cornflakes	Total cereal
French fries	Vanilla wafers

Maximal (Glycemic Index >85)

Dried dates	Instant mashed potatoes
French baguettes	Instant rice

rice or pearl barley to your next soup, stew, or casserole; add whole oats to cookies and other desserts; and if you like to bake, try replacing half the amount of white flour with whole-grain flour. Not only will the food taste great, you'll know that everyone eating it is getting a little longevity boost. You can also switch from white breads to 100 percent whole wheat, from refined cold cereals to whole-grain cereals, and from soda crackers to whole-grain wheat and rye crackers.

Whole-grain foods, including everything from a tasty array of whole-wheat pastas to long-grain rice pilaf mixes, are no longer specialty items for the very health-conscious shoppers with hours of time on their hands to seek them out. They are readily available, mass-marketed items accessible to everyone willing to take a few moments to notice what they're buying and eating. It is easy to shop and eat well, and the longevity benefits are tremendous.

The following list contains suggestions to help ensure that you get this basic healthy food group into your Longevity Diet.

Whole Grains, Legumes, and Other Carbohydrates

Barley: pearl, pot, or Scotch

Beans: black, cannellini, chickpeas (garbanzos), green, haricot, kidney, lima, pinto, soybeans

Bran: muffins, cereals, raw flakes

Breads: whole-wheat, multi-grain, rye, oat

Buckwheat: pancakes, kasha, muffins

Cereals: whole-grain, whole-wheat, wheat-berry, oat, bran, wheat germ, puffed rice, kasha

Crackers (whole grain)

Lentils: soup, dip

Oats: oatmeal, oatmeal cookies, oat cereals

Pasta: (whole-grain) linguini, spaghetti, rigatoni, macaroni

Peas: Chinese, split, black-eyed

Popcorn (unbuttered)

Rice: brown, wild

Tortillas (corn)

Tortilla chips (baked)

Whole-wheat couscous

Michele R. had always been tall and thin. In the sixth grade, the boys teased her and called her "Beanstalk." In college, those same boys practically killed themselves to get a date with her. Never a fan of real exercise, Michele enjoyed an occasional game of tennis and maybe a walk on the beach, and *all* her girlfriends hated her for being able to eat whatever she wanted and never gain an ounce.

But after age forty-six, things began to change. Usually full of energy, Michele started feeling tired a lot—especially after eating. And although she had gained only a pound or two since high school, her clothes didn't seem to fit her in the same way—pants and skirts felt tighter in the waist, tops seemed snug, and she just couldn't wait to change into her sweats at the end of the day. It got to the point that Michele felt so exhausted after dinner, she could hardly keep her eyes open or carry on a conversation. Because she attributed these changes to getting older, Michele finally contacted me at the UCLA Center on Aging and came into the clinic to discuss her tiredness and other symptoms she was experiencing.

After an in-depth discussion, it became clear that Michele had been eating a diet high in carbohydrates—many of them with a high glycemic index—and very little meat and other proteins. This diet was likely causing her blood sugar levels to spike sharply as she ate, and then come crashing down quickly afterward—leaving her feeling tired and depleted. Not only was this blood-glucose roller coaster bad for her heart and longevity, it was leading to weight gain around the abdomen, which was setting her up to develop insulin resistance and possibly adult-onset diabetes. Also, since the protein in her diet was insufficient, Michele may not have been getting enough essential amino acids, which make up the body's cells and the enzymes that keep those cells functioning.

I suggested that Michele eat a combination of all three healthy food groups: fruits and vegetables; proteins, lean meats, and healthy fats; and whole grains—in correct and healthy portions throughout the day. I also mentioned that to remain healthy, strong, and young-looking—as well as to get those clothes to fit like they used to—she should be sure to exercise regularly.

Three Days on the Longevity Diet

The proven benefits of each of the three food groups overlap. Fish and nuts not only contain protein and omega-3 fats, they are also good sources of antioxidant vitamins; many whole grains possess potent antioxidants, as well as some protein, fiber, and other nutrients; olive and other vegetable oils contain not only omega-3 fats, but also vitamin E antioxidants. The Longevity Diet makes it easy to combine these food groups to stay fit, trim, and healthy for the long haul, while still indulging in those *cheat eats* we may want to pamper ourselves with once in a while.

To get a better idea of how the diet works, here are the first three days that Shirley I. followed. Although she dropped two pounds during her first couple of weeks on the diet, Shirley did not set out to lose weight. Her goal was to feel healthier and stronger, look better, and reap the quality longevity benefits.

Recipes for menu suggestions marked with an asterisk (*) can be found in Appendix 1.

DAY ONE

Shirley drank a fresh, cool glass of water upon waking up.

Breakfast
¾–1 cup whole-oat oatmeal topped with 1 teaspoon brown sugar
½ cup lowfat (or nonfat) milk
½ grapefruit
Cup of coffee
Vitamin supplements: 1 multivitamin and 1 vitamin C (500 mg)

(The oatmeal—whole grain—*stars* in this meal.)

Midmorning Snack
½ cup lowfat cottage cheese, plus 1 tablespoon raisins mixed in
½ banana
Sparkling juice (1 part fruit juice plus 2 parts soda water, served
 over ice)

Lunch
Chef salad with mixed greens and sliced vegetables, 2 ounces
 sliced chicken, 1 ounce sliced lowfat Swiss cheese, 1 sliced egg
 white, tossed with olive oil vinaigrette dressing
2 whole-grain crackers
Sliced pear
Iced tea

(The chef salad meal *costars* vegetables and protein.)

Afternoon Snack
1 cup tomato soup or juice
1 ounce roasted almonds
Soda water with lemon

Dinner
Iceberg lettuce wedge with Roquefort Dressing*
Grilled 6-ounce salmon filet with herbs and lemon slices
½ cup wild rice
Steamed broccoli
Strawberry Sorbet*
Glass of white wine, ice water

(Salmon filet gives protein the *starring* role.)

Nighttime Snack
Frozen nonfat yogurt

DAY TWO

A refreshing glass of water.

Breakfast
Raisin-Bran Muffins* spread with ricotta cheese and real-fruit jam
½ cup fresh blueberries (frozen are good, too!)
Coffee
Vitamin supplements

(Whole grains *star*.)

Midmorning Snack
Bag of raw vegetables: celery/red bell pepper/tomatoes
1 ounce string cheese

Lunch
3-ounce tuna sandwich on whole-wheat bread, with lettuce and
    tomato (light mayo)
Crisp apple
Soda water with lemon

(Vegetables/fruits and whole grains share *star* billing, backed by a
    small amount of protein from the tuna in this healthy cross-
    trained meal.)

Afternoon Snack
Peach slices topped with ⅓ cup cottage cheese and a tablespoon
    of chopped almonds
Soda water with lemon

Dinner
6-ounce grilled chicken breast with herbs
Cheesy Pesto with Pasta* (side serving)
Steamed carrots
Apple Crumble à la Mode*
Glass of red wine, ice water

(Protein *stars.*)

Nighttime Snack
Frozen fruit-juice bar

DAY THREE

Wake-up water.

Breakfast
Vegetable omelet (use 1whole egg plus 2 or 3 egg whites)
½ cup fresh or frozen blueberries
Coffee
Vitamin supplements: 1 multivitamin and 1 vitamin C (500 mg)

(Omelet—protein—*stars* in this meal.)

Midmorning Snack
½ cup nonfat plain or flavored yogurt with 1 tablespoon raisins
Tea (green has the most antioxidant value)

Lunch
Bowl of chicken soup (with white meat and vegetables)
Spinach salad with chopped apple and walnuts, vinaigrette
    dressing

Orange sections
Iced tea

(Fruits and vegetables *star*.)

Afternoon Snack
Raw vegetable sticks with 2 tablespoons of peanut butter (lowfat
  preferred)
Iced tea

Dinner
Tomato, avocado, and sweet onion salad; olive oil and vinegar
Mixed Seafood and Linguini* using ¾ cup whole-wheat linguini
Steamed asparagus spears
Cheat Eat: Slice of devil's food cake
Arnold Palmer on ice (½ iced tea and ½ lemonade)

(Seafood—protein—*stars* in this meal.)

Nighttime Snack
Sliced fresh apple with cinnamon

Losing Weight

Although many people lose pounds without even trying when
they begin the Longevity Diet, others who wish to drop pounds
more quickly can make some of the following modifications to the
diet:

- Cut back on your carbohydrates and eat more lean and nonfat protein "starring" meals, along with vegetables, salad, and
  fruit for dessert.
- Cut out alcoholic beverages and *all* cheat eats.

- Limit your servings. Recent research shows that people eat less when they are served smaller portions.
- Remember to eat your healthy snacks between meals, so you don't get overly hungry and overeat later.
- Be sure to drink at least eight glasses of water a day.
- Increase your amount of exercise, especially the cardiovascular component. Also, keep in mind that strength training helps build lean body mass, which raises your metabolism and helps you burn more calories and therefore lose more weight (see Essential 6).

This will serve as your *quick start* diet program, which should give you a greater sense of control, after which you can begin to add some more of the healthy whole grains, alcohol if you desire, and even the occasional cheat eat. You can stay on the weight reduction program as long as you need to, but unless you have more than ten pounds to lose, you should be able to transition to the regular Longevity Diet within four weeks and enjoy the benefits of a lifetime of delicious and healthy eating.

Getting Started

When preparing to begin the Longevity Diet, it's a good idea to take stock of your pantry and refrigerator, and make a shopping list of the foods you'll need for your first week of healthy longevity eating. Planning a few days' meals in advance will help.

By stocking up on some basics such as fresh fruits, vegetables, and herbs, lean meats, fish, brown rice, olive oil, vinegar, whole-wheat bread and pasta, cheeses, eggs, nonfat yogurt, and milk, you will be ready to make just about any of the easy meals and recipes in this book, and many other delicious concoctions you come up with yourself.

Many people find it helpful to plan their cross-training meals and chart their progress using a daily food chart or diary. Make some copies of the following blank chart to help ensure that your meals and snacks include at least two of the three healthy food groups. Place an asterisk (*) next to the food that *stars* in each of your meals.

Day _____	Fruits/Vegetables	Proteins/Fats	Carbohydrates
Breakfast			
Snack			
Lunch			
Snack			
Dinner			
Snack			

Following the Longevity Diet

- Eat the foods you like the most from the following food groups. Each food group can *star* in up to two meals per day.
  - Antioxidant fruits and vegetables
  - Proteins, lean meats, and healthy fats
  - Whole grains, legumes, and other carbohydrates
- Use mindful awareness to focus on how your body feels before, during, and after eating to help you gauge portion size and know when you've had enough.
- Occasionally indulge in a small portion of your favorite cheat eats.
- Drink at least eight glasses of water throughout the day.
- Enjoy two to three healthy between-meal snacks a day.
- Avoid excessive salts, bad fats, and high glycemic-index carbohydrates.
- If you wish to lose weight, cut back on carbohydrates, alcohol, and cheat eats until you reach your goal.

Essential 8

Modern Medicine for Feeling and Looking Younger

By medicine, life may be prolonged . . .
— WILLIAM SHAKESPEARE

Medical breakthroughs in the last decade are promising to keep us alive and healthy longer than any generation before us. Within our lifetime, living past the age of one hundred may become commonplace. Modern medical technologies such as heart transplants and Lasik eye surgery have already become routine procedures. Complex neuroimaging techniques—windows into what used to be the hidden, secret workings of the body—have led to screening tests and new surgical methods that allow us to control and often beat major killers such as colon cancer and heart disease. More effective medicines with fewer side effects have added years to our lives. Soon, we may be able to manage Alzheimer's disease in the same way that we deal with high blood pressure today—through simple tests and preventive medicine.

This *Longevity Bible* Essential covers the newest medical techniques for *staying, feeling,* and *looking* young. We'll look at breakthrough interventions such as new cures for cancer, ways to fire up our libido, and the latest cosmetic innovations aimed at keeping us looking eternally youthful.

With the mapping of the human genome, we can now expect more targeted therapies that take into account an individual's specific genetic profile. Stem cells have the remarkable potential to develop into almost any cell type in the body, and scientists may eventually be able to grow these primitive cells to replace diseased ones, and even entire organs. Swedish scientists recently used adult human stem cells to generate functioning brain cells.

Nanotechnology is a new field that builds objects and substances one atom or molecule at a time. It is a form of molecular engineering that will lead to a manufacturing revolution. Scientists have already used nanotechnologies to build minute robots powered by the beat of a single heart cell. These could one day lead to micro-robotic heart muscles that would keep our hearts beating long beyond their previous capacity.

With obesity rapidly becoming one of the greatest health threats of the twenty-first century, scientists have developed an injectable hormone that literally switches off a person's appetite. In initial tests, it enabled people to lose over five pounds a month without trying. An implantable heart defibrillator is also being developed to provide an electric shock to the heart muscle to reset its rhythm in the event of a heart attack, which could save millions of lives each year.

Thanks to the latest in medical innovations, we should all start planning to look and feel younger—well into our eighties, nineties, and beyond. New treatments can make us *look* younger in a multitude of ways—from smoother skin to more hair—as well as *feel* younger, with greater mobility and improved joint function. We can now improve our quality of life by boosting our libidos and energy levels. With the wide array of medicines, treatments, and procedures becoming available, it is essential to become an informed consumer, choosing and monitoring your *medical portfolio* wisely—just as you would your financial portfolio. Knowing how to effectively use new medical technologies is a key to this quality longevity essential.

Living Longer

Only a generation ago, cancer was almost always fatal. Now there is not only earlier detection, but there are also more effective treatments and sometimes cures. Cancer and heart disease, however, are still the leading causes of death in the United States. In the most common form of heart disease, the coronary arteries—vessels that supply blood and nutrients to heart muscles—become clogged from the buildup of fatty plaque over time. For people with severe blockage of coronary arteries, bypass surgery or angioplasty can be lifesaving. In bypass surgery, the diseased coronary arteries are replaced by healthy blood vessels from the leg, arm, or chest. A less invasive alternative for some patients is angioplasty. In this procedure, the cardiologist inserts a balloon-tipped catheter into a large blood vessel in the arm or leg and guides it to the blocked coronary artery, where it is inflated to stretch the artery. A wire mesh tube, or *stent*, is left in place to keep the artery open.

With proper treatment, chronic and fatal conditions such as high blood pressure or high cholesterol pose less of a risk. In a study of patients with only mild elevations in blood pressure, treatment with antihypertensive drugs increased life expectancy by two to three years. Other studies have found that lowering blood pressure by only five points reduces the risk of stroke by an estimated 34 percent and heart disease by 21 percent.

A recent study found that taking a statin (cholesterol-lowering) drug within the first twenty-four hours after a heart attack can decrease the risk of death by 50 percent. Scientists have also found that statin drugs can reduce deaths from advanced heart failure by as much as 55 percent. By lowering blood cholesterol levels, statins keep fatty deposits from building up and eventually blocking circulation. The drugs may also protect the heart by reducing inflammation, which plays a role in heart failure.

Over the past decade, the total death rate from cancer has dropped by more than 12 percent in the United States. The greatest declines—accounting for over fifty-five thousand lives saved—were found in prostate and lung cancer in men, breast cancer in women, and colon cancer in both sexes. Earlier detection of prostate cancer is now possible through prostate-specific antigen (PSA) screening, a simple blood test.

A new cancer treatment, androgen blockade, can essentially beat cancer long enough for some patients to live normally and eventually die from unrelated causes. Better treatments for breast cancer, such as the drug tamoxifen and other chemotherapies, are improving survival rates, along with widespread use of mammography for early detection. And invasive interventions are not always necessary to save lives. Recent reports published in the *New England Journal of Medicine* found that lumpectomy followed by radiation can be just as effective as complete mastectomy.

Colorectal cancer is the second leading cause of cancer deaths. If diagnosed early through colonoscopy, it is often curable with surgery. Risk for the disease increases after age fifty, particularly for those with a family history. Less than a third of Americans over age fifty have had a colonoscopy. Although the preparation can be uncomfortable, this detection procedure takes only about a half hour and can be a lifesaver.

Feeling Younger

Besides extending life expectancy, medical interventions—drugs, surgeries, and alternative treatments—can improve our quality of life. Many patients are taking advantage of new technologies that allow them to monitor their own symptoms electronically. Wireless armbands can now take blood-sugar readings and beam them directly to physicians. "Smart" scales can wire your weight to the clinic and display back to you your doctor's follow-up questions and answers.

MANAGING MEDICINES

Numerous medications have become available to treat symptoms of severe diseases, as well as common and annoying age-related complaints. However, when we take too many drugs, we may get into trouble with side effects. Managing medicines can be a challenge—especially for older people, who tend to take more medicines throughout the day.

When Nancy G. finally got to her mother's apartment, she knew they were already late for her mom's doctor's appointment. She frantically searched for Mom's daily blood-pressure chart—it was on the counter, hiding behind the insulin injection kit. Nancy called out to Mom to make sure she got her medications together—the doctor had specifically asked her to bring all her drugs to the appointment so he could make sure that her medicines weren't worsening her memory. When her mother came into the kitchen carrying two large shopping bags, Nancy once again felt frustrated by her mom's forgetfulness. "Mother, I told you that we don't have time to get to the mall today and return those gifts." But when Nancy looked *inside* the bags, she saw they were entirely filled with medicine bottles, samples, and prescriptions from various doctors. And these were just the drugs her mom was *currently* taking.

The average older person takes more than a half dozen prescription medicines at any one time, and the more medicines a person takes, the greater the possibility for side effects to occur. A recent study found that one out of every four older adults receives at least one inappropriate or unnecessary medicine. Also, many people still use older medicines they began taking several years ago that are often less safe than newer drugs developed for the same purpose.

As we get older, the receptors throughout our bodies become more sensitive to the effects of drugs, increasing the possibility of side effects at much lower doses. Also, our bodies become less efficient in breaking down and eliminating medicines, so that over time we may accumulate higher blood levels of drugs. This can lead to new or increased side effects, as well as interactions with other drugs that we hadn't experienced in the past. Even over-the-counter and herbal remedies, which many people consider safe, can sometimes have undesirable or dangerous side effects. For instance, someone taking ginkgo, aspirin, and vitamin E together might experience unexpected bruising and excessive bleeding. Due to the changes in our bodies, doctors caring for older individuals often prescribe drugs in low doses initially and then slowly increase them as needed, to minimize any potential negative reactions.

Many medications have anticholinergic side effects, meaning that they oppose the actions of drugs prescribed for memory loss, thereby worsening memory. Over-the-counter antihistamines such as Benadryl can have this effect, particularly on older people. Drugs prescribed for anxiety—such as Xanax, Valium, or Librium—are frequently overused and can cause sedation and memory impairment, as well as an increased risk of falling. Drugs used to regulate heart rate or treat high blood pressure can make blood vessels less taut and decrease the heart's ability to pump blood. Since our vascular tone diminishes as we age anyway, medicines that aggravate this problem can lead to falls, head trauma, and other complications, so they should be taken with care.

Alan F.'s wife kept nagging him to go back to the doctor for his routine checkup but he just didn't have the time—the hotel business had gotten so dog-eat-dog lately and there were so many young upstarts vying to secure management jobs like his. Besides, last time the doctor had put him on blood-pressure pills that made him so sleepy he'd hardly been able to keep his eyes open past 9 p.m. He knew his wife thought he just didn't want to be intimate with her anymore, but it wasn't true. He was simply too exhausted every night to deal with it. Unfortunately, Alan's growing marital stress at home, on top of the stress he had at work all day, wasn't doing his blood pressure any favors—even *with* the medication. Alan was beginning to feel depressed and considered asking his doctor about trying an antidepressant. But then he read that they could have negative sexual performance side effects, and that was the last thing he needed.

When Alan finally did go in for his exam and explain all this, his physician switched him to a different blood-pressure medicine. The doctor told Alan to call sooner about any drug side effects that might arise when starting a new treatment. In fact, the doctor noted that the first blood-pressure medicine Alan had taken was occasionally associated with decreased libido. Alan wondered if he could get a doctor's note about that to give his wife.

With the new medicine change, Alan's energy and enthusiasm returned, along with his libido, and soon his depression lifted. The doctor had even given him some Viagra samples to try, but Alan didn't need them. His renewed vitality improved his outlook at work, as well. Alan's wife seemed happier, too, for some reason.

When discussing possible drug interactions with your doctor, be sure to mention any over-the-counter medicines you take, as well as supplements and foods you eat that may increase or decrease the effects of your medicines. Some drugs interact with grapefruit juice, which can increase the medicine's effects and the risk for side effects. Be sure you truly need a particular drug, and that your doctor is aware of all the medicines you currently take. This is especially important if you are under the care of more than one doctor. Pharmacists can be helpful in answering questions regarding drug interactions, as well. For more information on specific drug interactions check the Web site *www.druginteractioncenter.org*.

It is important *not* to stop taking prescribed medications on your own. Researchers at the University of Michigan found that when middle-aged and older people stop their prescription medicines without consulting their doctors, 32 percent experience a serious decline in health.

The U.S. Food and Drug Administration (FDA) provides an Internet guide (*www.fda.gov/oc/buyonline/default.htm*) describing the risks of buying medicines and related products on the Internet. Dangers are everywhere on the Web, including contaminated or counterfeit products, incorrect dosages, expired medicines, illegal uses of medicines, and other problems. The guide helps consumers with clues for differentiating fake Internet sites from legitimate ones. Several points to keep in mind include finding out whether or not the online pharmacy is licensed and provides access to a registered pharmacist, being cautious of sites based in foreign countries, avoiding online pharmacy sites that let you get medicines without a doctor's prescription, and making sure the site provides an actual street address and phone number—an e-mail address is not enough.

BLOOD PRESSURE—STAYING LOW

Hypertension affects approximately 60 percent of the population, a 10 percent increase in just the past decade. Under high pressure, stiffened blood vessels can rupture, and may cause cerebrovascular disease involving blood leakage into the brain tissue, and eventual stroke. A stroke is often defined as the death of brain cells, resulting in a loss of physical or mental function, or both. When tissue death occurs in the heart, it pumps less effectively, which can cause heart failure or death.

Contrary to popular belief, people cannot tell if their blood pressure is high, and most patients with high blood pressure have no symptoms. Yet high blood pressure is easily detected with a blood-pressure cuff and stethoscope at your doctor's office or with a home device, and it's effectively treated with a variety of antihypertensive medicines. The most effective strategy combines medicine and lifestyle changes—avoiding cigarettes and overeating and getting enough exercise are crucial, as well as staying away from the salt shaker. Regular exercise and a healthy diet can sometimes even eliminate the need for medicines.

A new study suggests that what was previously considered normal blood pressure may not be so normal. The current guidelines set normal systolic blood pressure (when the heart is contracting) at less than 140 millimeters, and the diastolic (when the heart is relaxed) at less than 90. In this new study, patients had normal blood pressure, but were still at risk for heart problems. Those who received antihypertensive drugs had mild drops in blood pressure and a 30 percent decline in heart attacks, strokes, or hospitalizations for chest pain.

KEEPING BONES STRONG

More than ten million Americans, mostly women, suffer from osteoporosis, which essentially means that the bones get porous, brittle, and weak. Hip fractures are a major risk when bones weaken, and each year the number of women suffering from hip fractures exceeds the combined number who get heart attacks, strokes, and breast cancer. Age, estrogen deficiency, family history, and smoking are risk factors, and diagnosis is made using a special bone density scan called a DEXA (dual energy X-ray absorptiometry) scan, which is recommended for all women over age sixty-five, regardless of their risk.

To keep bones healthy, the National Academy of Sciences and the National Osteoporosis Foundation recommend daily calcium intakes of 1,000 to 1,200 milligrams for adult men and women, preferably from food, but also from supplements, if necessary. Between four hundred and eight hundred international units (IUs) of Vitamin D also are needed to help the body to absorb calcium.

Several medicines are available to treat osteoporosis, once it is diagnosed, which can greatly reduce the risk for bone fractures. Estrogen replacement therapy has been shown to significantly decrease this risk, and the bisphosphonates alendronate (Fosamax) and risedronate (Actonel) can substantially reduce the risk of both hip and spine fractures.

Calcitonin (Miacalcin) can be taken either by injection or through nose spray and is effective in increasing bone density, but mainly in the spine. It has been found to reduce pain from compression fractures of the spine. Selective estrogen receptor modulators augment bone strength without negative effects on the breasts or the uterus, but they can increase the risk of strokes.

Lifestyle has a large impact on hip-fracture risk. Routine weight-bearing, stretching, and strengthening exercises (see Essential 6) will improve muscle and bone strength, as well as balance. Seniors who begin a weight-lifting regimen not only help to keep their bones young and strong, but can actually improve bone density and eventually feel ten or more years younger. A recent study of forty-six pairs of identical twins found that moderate alcohol intake was associated with greater bone density, which reduces the risk for fractures.

PREVENTING AND CONTROLLING DIABETES

Approximately eighteen million Americans suffer from diabetes. Their bodies have trouble metabolizing sugar or glucose, and often pills or insulin injections are needed to get sugar from the blood into the body's cells to maintain the chemical reactions that sustain consciousness and life. Diet, weight control, and exercise are the most effective strategies for preventing and controlling this condition, but if oral medications are needed to lower blood-sugar levels, several are safe and effective. Sulfonylurea drugs stimulate the pancreas to produce and release more insulin. Another option is to use newer drugs known as meglitinides, which work quickly and can be safer.

Pharmaceutical companies have been pushing to develop drugs to prevent diabetes symptoms before people develop the full-blown disease. Metformin, marketed as Glucophage, as well as rosiglitazone (Avandia), treat diabetes symptoms, and studies show that such drugs may help prevent the disease in some people at risk. A recent report from the journal *Lancet* found that a group of overweight patients at risk for diabetes did significantly better than the placebo group, on a new drug known as rimonabant, which was effective in helping them to lose weight, improve insulin response, and lower blood cholesterol.

CHOLESTEROL BUSTING

For many people, blood cholesterol levels creep upward over the years and, if untreated, may result in heart disease and stroke. Risk factors for developing high cholesterol include diabetes, smoking, high blood pressure, lack of exercise, and obesity. Quitting smoking, losing weight, dieting, and getting regular exercise all contribute to lower cholesterol levels.

For years, doctors have been telling us to control our cholesterol levels, especially the LDL, or "bad" cholesterol. A new report from the National Cholesterol Education Program updates earlier guidelines setting LDL goals for high-risk people to 70 (down from 100). These new levels mean that an estimated forty million Americans should be taking some action to lower their cholesterol, including taking statin drugs.

Recent research suggests that some patients should be on cholesterol-lowering drugs regardless of their blood cholesterol levels. The American College of Physicians recently recommended that all diabetics age fifty-five years or older should be on statin drugs, as should younger diabetics with other risk factors such as heart disease or high blood pressure. The guidelines stemmed from a review of studies finding that statin drugs reduced the rate of heart attacks and other cardiac problems by approximately 23 percent in diabetics with cardiac risks.

The power of statins appears to benefit other illnesses. In laboratory studies, statin drugs inhibit the growth of colon-cancer cells, and a recent study of nearly four thousand volunteers found that at least five years of statin use was associated with a 47 percent reduction in the risk of colorectal cancer. Although these studies are encouraging, doctors are not yet recommending statins as preventive treatments for cancer until additional investigations confirm these initial findings. Other research suggests that statins may delay the onset of Alzheimer's disease or delay its progression.

KEEP YOUR JOINTS MOVING

Osteoarthritis is the most common form of arthritis and can be a debilitating progressive disease. There is no cure, but treatments have advanced considerably in recent years. The big push in therapy has been to augment treatments that reduce pain and increase mobility with therapies that interfere with the actual disease progression. Most current treatment strategies include medicines along with physical therapy, exercise, weight management, and, as a last resort, surgery.

Nonsteroidal anti-inflammatory drugs (NSAIDs) relieve pain and fight inflammation and are available over the counter or by prescription. Examples include ibuprofen (Advil, Motrin, and others) and naproxen sodium (Aleve). These drugs do have potential side effects, such as bleeding, ulcers, and liver and kidney damage. Newer anti-inflammatory drugs known as COX-2 inhibitors (e.g., Celebrex, Bextra, and Vioxx) were originally thought to be safer as far as causing stomach bleeding, but potential cardiac side effects led manufacturers to take several of them off the market.

Over-the-counter Tylenol (acetaminophen) can reduce pain as effectively as NSAIDs, but taking more than the recommended dose may damage the liver. Another approach involves the use of lidocaine patches that are applied to areas of pain, such as the back or the knee. A recent study presented at the American Pain Society found that such patches were as effective as the anti-inflammatory drug Celebrex. The lidocaine, which is similar to the novocaine injected to numb the gums during dental procedures, inhibits pain signals to the brain but does not cause numbness. The only potential side effect from the patches is minor skin irritation.

Surgical techniques for joint replacement—most often the knee or hip—have advanced considerably, and these are now often outpatient procedures that allow people to get back on their feet quickly. The surgeon removes the damaged joint and replaces it with a plastic or metal prosthesis. Many patients resume normal levels of activity and enjoy improved mobility and pain reduction.

ALZHEIMER'S DISE...
PREVENTION AND TREATMENT

Alzheimer's disease afflicts approximately five million Americans, and millions more suffer from mild cognitive impairment, which puts them at risk for developing the disease. Family members and friends also suffer as they watch patients gradually lose their memory and other cognitive functions. Recent research has shown that lifestyle choices can significantly lower the risk for developing the disease. Innovative medicines and vaccines that might delay its onset are under investigation.

Most of the currently available drugs to improve memory and other cognitive symptoms do so by enhancing the brain's level of acetylcholine, the chemical neurotransmitter that facilitates the passage of nerve impulses across synapses. The brains of Alzheimer's patients have a deficiency of acetylcholine, which can result from either impaired production or excess breakdown by enzymes called cholinesterases. Drugs such as Aricept, Exelon, and Razadyne inhibit these enzymes, so they are called "cholinesterase inhibitors."

Memantine, marketed as Namenda, works on the brain's NMDA (N-methyl-D-aspartate) receptors by blocking the chemical glutamate, which overstimulates these receptors, allowing too much calcium to enter cells, leading to cell destruction. Namenda has been approved for patients with moderate to severe Alzheimer's disease, but many clinicians find it effective in milder stages, as well. The drug is safe when used with a cholinesterase inhibitor drug such as Aricept, and initial studies show that the combination provides a greater benefit than using only one drug.

DOSING OF COMMONLY USED DRUGS FOR DEMENTIA

Drug	Start Dose	Highest Dose
Donepezil (Aricept)	5 mg, once a day	10 mg, once a day
Rivastigmine (Exelon)	1.5 mg, twice a day	6 mg, twice a day
Galantamine (Razadyne ER)	8 mg, once a day	24 mg, once a day
Memantine (Namenda)	5 mg, once a day	10 mg, twice a day

Alzheimer's patients who take these drugs need fewer medications for treating depression and behavior problems. They also remain at home and out of nursing homes longer than patients who do not take the medicines. These drugs not only improve memory and thinking, but can also reduce agitation and depression and can help with related illnesses, including vascular and Lewy Body Dementia. At UCLA, we are testing these drugs to see if they slow down brain aging in healthy people and possibly prevent Alzheimer's disease.

Scientists have found that the earlier the disease is recognized and treated, the better the outcome. In September 2004, the Centers for Medicare and Medicaid Services approved the use of positron emission tomography (PET) scans for Medicare reimbursement to assist doctors in better diagnosing Alzheimer's disease, in part so that the disease can be recognized and treated earlier. A recent study indicated that when Aricept was used in patients with mild cognitive impairment, it delayed the onset of Alzheimer's disease, as compared with a placebo.

At UCLA, our approach to Alzheimer's disease is to protect the brain before damage sets in—using several of the *Longevity Bible* Essentials. Our initial studies found that healthy volunteers ages thirty-five to seventy who spent just two weeks on a healthy lifestyle program, combining body fitness, mental aerobics, healthy diet, and stress reduction, experienced significant improvemen ciency in a key memory center where Alzheimer's strikes. In some people, memory scores improved percent—in just fourteen days—as if volunteers had subtracted two decades from their brain age.

Our scientific team at UCLA has developed a new way to use the PET scanner so that the physical evidence of Alzheimer's disease, the abnormal amyloid protein build-up, can be measured in the living patient, as opposed to the traditional method whereby Alzheimer's could be proven only after a patient died, through autopsy. Our research group has been able to spot these abnormal proteins using the new amyloid-PET scanner in people with only mild cognitive impairment, years before they are likely to develop Alzheimer's disease. This will allow doctors to initiate prevention strategies as soon as possible. Many companies are developing drugs and vaccines designed to disrupt the buildup of the amyloid proteins that begin accumulating in the brain's memory centers early in adulthood and may lead to Alzheimer's disease.

AVOIDING THE BLUES

An estimated 15 percent of the population develops a clinical depression at some point in their lives. When left untreated, patients experience not just emotional symptoms of sadness, loss of interest, and guilt, but also have physical symptoms, including weight loss, fatigue, and insomnia. Depressed people also tend to experience more physical pain. Professional treatment of the depression can alleviate both the physical and emotional symptoms. Many depressions involve more than one trigger or cause, with overlapping psychological and biological factors contributing. Regardless of the specific cause, patients who receive psychotherapy, antidepressant drugs, or both usually improve, even if their symptoms are severe.

One feature of depression—decreased ability to concentrate— seems to become more prominent as we age. Middle-aged and older people tend to emphasize these concentration difficulties and their depressions are often colored by memory complaints. Unfortunately, many people still consider depression to be a sign of character weakness, so they avoid seeking professional help or taking antidepressants. What those people often don't realize is that untreated depression can increase a person's risk for serious physical illness or even death, as well as raise the risk for suicide. The life-expectancy rate for patients whose depressions are properly treated and improved is twice that of those who do not receive adequate care.

Although all types of antidepressant drugs have been effective in relieving some symptoms of depression, the improved side effect profiles of the newer antidepressants, such as fluoxetine (Prozac), sertraline (Zoloft), citalopram (Celexa), or paroxetine (Paxil), to mention a few, have caused them to become preferred treatments over older medicines such as amitriptyline (Elavil) or imipramine (Tofranil). These older medicines can potentially worsen memory performance because of their anticholinergic side effects. Some also cause blood pressure drops that can cause people to fall when they get up too quickly.

It is best to start low and go slowly with antidepressant medicines, particularly when treating older people. Many primary-care physicians can treat depression quite effectively using antidepressants, but for a complicated and more severe depression, the expertise of a psychiatrist may be needed. A psychiatrist with additional geriatric training can offer the most sophisticated care for some depressed older patients.

PROTECTING VISION

As we age, vision tends to decline, and it often gets harder to read small print, whether it's in a newspaper or on a pillbox. To accommodate the millions of baby boomers with lower visual acuity, several publishers are now increasing the height and print size of their mass-market paperbacks. If you can't find your favorite novel with the right font size, corrective lenses are available in a variety of shapes and sizes.

Eye disease is also more likely as we age, but preventive measures—including sunglasses to block damaging ultraviolet light, getting enough antioxidant fruits and vegetables, or taking supplements such as vitamins A, C, and E—greatly reduce risks. Because diabetes and hypertension can lead to eye disease, a healthy diet and regular exercise are effective prevention strategies. Also, regular eye exams, including checks of eye pressure, are essential.

Approximately 50 percent of older adults get *cataracts* that cloud vision from damage to the lens. Vision often improves following cataract surgery to replace the cloudy lens with a clear plastic one. Laser or conventional surgery also may benefit *macular degeneration*, a common eye disorder in older people that causes hazy vision and a central blind spot from the breakdown of light-sensitive cells in the central part of the eye's retina.

Glaucoma causes vision loss in approximately three million Americans. Excess fluid elevates eye pressure and damages the optic nerve, a bundle of nerve fibers at the back of the eye. With early detection, treatment, and monitoring, blind spots and eventual blindness usually can be prevented. One of the most prescribed eye drops for lowering eye pressure is a prostaglandin analogue known as latanoprost (Xalatan). Research has found that after two years of treatment with Xalatan, only 7 percent of patients require additional glaucoma medicine or need to switch to another medicine. Other commonly used alternatives are bimatoprost (Lumigan), travoprost (Travatan), and timolol (Timoptic). If eyedrops alone don't bring down eye pressure, an oral medication may be added, such as a carbonic anhydrase inhibitor. Laser treatments and conventional surgery are other options that may be necessary to lower eye pressure.

HEARING WELL

The blaring rock concerts some of us enjoyed in our youth were lots of fun, but the exposure to those high decibel levels can catch up with us eventually. Approximately one third or more of older adults have some degree of hearing loss, and exposure to loud noises is one of the most common contributing factors. It is best to avoid exposure to extreme sounds by either using ear protection or just not going there. Although hearing aids can help many forms of hearing loss, only about one out of every five people who could benefit actually use them. A doctor who specializes in hearing can help guide you to the best intervention. The wide range of hearing aids available include cochlear implants, small devices that are surgically implanted under the skin, behind the ear. A recent study found that such implants significantly improve not just the comprehension of speech, but overall quality of life, as well.

LIBIDO BOOSTERS

Individuals differ in their sexual needs and desires throughout life. As people age, the hormone testosterone declines in both men and women, which may diminish sexual desire. Also, physical illnesses, depression, hormonal changes associated with menopause, and some medications can reduce sex drive. Chronic pain can also limit sexual activity, so careful timing of pain medicines can make sex more enjoyable and satisfying. Despite such age-related changes, several treatments are safe and effective and help millions to continue to have fulfilling sex throughout their lives.

Female Enhancers. After menopause, hormonal changes may diminish sex drive in women, but many women find they can get a libido boost with estrogen replacement therapy. Although it isn't clear that estrogen replacement has a direct effect on libido, it has been shown to help those who experience pain associated with intercourse. Because of concern about long-term side effects from estrogen pills or patches, many have turned to locally applied estrogen creams. These creams also help reduce vaginal dryness, which often hinders post-menopausal sex drive. Sexual activity itself increases vaginal blood flow, which stimulates lubrication.

Testosterone is usually thought of as a male sex hormone, but women also have small amounts in their bodies, produced primarily by their ovaries. After menopause, testosterone levels will decline, which can lower the drive for sex. Although not yet approved by the FDA, the testosterone patch has been found to improve sexual desire in women with low libido. In a recent controlled study, the testosterone patch increased sexual desire and satisfaction in women who had had their ovaries surgically removed. The patch is usually applied to the lower stomach area and is changed twice each week.

Male Enhancers. You've probably seen the TV ads showing a middle-aged couple walking hand-in-hand on the beach, or a man and woman relaxing in a hot tub for two. With the introduction of Cialis and Levitra, Viagra no longer has the corner on the erectile dysfunction market. The clinical impression is that all three drugs are similar in effectiveness, though Cialis claims to last about thirty-six hours—you can't be *too* ready if the time is right—compared to about four hours for the others.

Doctors who prescribe these drugs should first check for high blood pressure, diabetes, and other medical conditions. These medicines should not be used more than once daily, and should never be used in combination with nitroglycerine, because it can be lethal. Recent rare reports of sudden vision loss in some men who took Viagra have led the manufacturer to change its labeling, but whether the drug directly causes this side effect has not been substantiated.

SUPPLEMENTS AND HORMONES

People of all ages spend billions each year on dietary supplements. Despite the numerous dramatic promises of a better sex life, a more muscular physique, or a cure for a variety of illnesses, the safety and the effectiveness of many of these products often fall short of the claims. As we get older, we are more inclined to use supplements: The majority of people age sixty and older currently take some kind of supplement.

False claims have been a problem for many years. Back in 1994, the Dietary Supplement and Health Education Act set forth the only standards for manufacturers, who are responsible for the truthfulness of label claims. Manufacturers must have evidence that supports their claims, but the FDA provides no guidelines for validating that evidence, nor does it require manufacturers to submit that evidence.

Of course, many of the claims are enticing. The supplement called conjugated linoleic acid, or CLA, has been touted as effective for weight loss and muscle building, and as a preventive treatment for heart disease, cancer, and diabetes. Although some initial studies were interesting, there is no definitive evidence to back the claims. Also, many herbal sex aids sold in magazines and on the Internet are, at best, ineffective and, at worst, dangerous.

To prove that a supplement really works for a specific illness or condition, scientists need to complete a "double-blind" clinical trial. To do this, they need to compare their supplement to an inactive placebo, and make sure neither the investigators nor the study subjects are aware of which pill is the active compound and which is the placebo. Most supplements don't get this kind of supportive evidence, so be cautious.

When deciding on which form or brand of supplement to take, consumers need accurate information about the level of evidence on the supplement's safety, effectiveness, and dosage. A knowledgeable pharmacist or physician can often help. Other resources include the National Center for Complementary and Alternative Medicine (*nccam.nih.gov*) and the Natural Medicines Comprehensive Database (*www.naturaldatabase.com*). Dietary supplements are available in most food and drug stores nationwide.

Vitamins. Because of vitamin E's ability to neutralize free radicals—unstable molecules that may damage the genetic material of healthy cells—it has been studied and used to help prevent such age-related conditions as heart disease, cancer, and Alzheimer's. This fat-soluble vitamin boosts the immune system and helps keep eyes and skin healthy. The average individual gets about 10 to 15 IUs of vitamin E each day from their diet. For patients with Alzheimer's disease, one previous study found that 2000 IUs of daily vitamin E delayed functional decline.

Recently, the Women's Health Study did *not* find that 600 IUs of daily vitamin E prevented heart attacks, stroke, or cancers of the lungs, breast, or colon. It *did* find, however, that vitamin E increased the risk of heart attack in women over age sixty-five. Another recent study from Johns Hopkins University School of Medicine found that people taking 400 IUs or more of vitamin E each day had a higher death rate than those on placebo. Because the deaths generally occurred in study subjects who also suffered from chronic diseases, the results may not apply to healthy people. Although many other studies have found vitamin E to be safe, this controversial Johns Hopkins study has left many doctors waiting for further evidence before routinely recommending high doses of vitamin E. People who want to play it safe can stop taking vitamin E for the time being, or drop their daily dose to less than 400 IUs.

Vitamin C is an antioxidant that can be taken safely at 500 to 1,000 mg daily. Like other antioxidant vitamins, it may not only protect brain health, but may also defend against some forms of cancer and diabetes, as well as increase immune defenses against colds and viruses. The Longevity Diet (see Essential 7) recommends a daily 500 mg vitamin C supplement.

Coenzyme Q_{10} is an antioxidant that has been used to treat age-related memory loss and to slow the progression of Alzheimer's and Parkinson's disease, although definitive scientific evidence of its effectiveness is limited. Coenzyme Q_{10} should be taken with caution, because it can interact with medicines used to treat heart failure, diabetes, and kidney or liver problems.

A daily multivitamin is a good idea because, as we age, our bodies lose their ability to absorb many vitamins and nutrients. Vitamin B_{12} absorption is a particular challenge: 20 percent of people age sixty and older, and 40 percent of those over age eighty, lose some of their ability to absorb vitamin B_{12}. The antioxidant B vitamin folate, or folic acid, protects us from developing strokes and heart disease. Some studies have shown that when Alzheimer's victims are treated with high doses of vitamin B_{12} or folate, their memory abilities improve. A large-scale seven-year study found that high doses of vitamins C and E, beta carotene, and zinc caused a 25 percent slowing in the progressive visual loss associated with macular degeneration. If the estimated eight million Americans over age fifty-five who are at risk for this disease took this combination of vitamins, 300,000 fewer individuals would lose their vision in the next five years. The Longevity Diet (see Essential 7) recommends a daily multivitamin.

It's important to avoid the potential toxic effects of unnecessary vitamin megadoses. This may be a particular problem with vitamins A, D, E, and K, which get stored in fat and can hang around in our bodies for weeks, months, or longer. If you're unsure about how much of any vitamin to take, check with your doctor or pharmacist.

Curcumin. This yellow spice found in curry powder also gives mustard its bright yellow color. Curcumin has been used for many years as an herbal remedy in India. Laboratory studies have demonstrated its anti-inflammatory and antioxidant effects, which may protect brain cells and help prevent cancer. Evidence suggests its potential benefits for colorectal, breast, prostate, and lung cancer. India—where curried food is so popular—has one of the world's lowest rates of Alzheimer's disease. The frequency of the disease in adults in India ages seventy to seventy-nine years is more than four times less than the frequency in the United States for the same age group. Curcumin is currently under study as a treatment for mild memory loss and Alzheimer's disease.

Omega-3 Supplements. Because of their potential for reducing the risk of cardiovascular disease, stroke, and Alzheimer's disease, omega-3 fats, such as docosahexaenoic acid or DHA, are available as supplements. Omega-3 fats minimize inflammation that can damage brain and heart cells, and have an antioxidant effect that fights against free radicals, which can further injure cells. Recent studies suggest that omega-3-rich supplements may help a person's mood, as well as their memory. These supplements usually contain fish oil, which is sensitive to light and to air oxidation. Make sure that you purchase the supplements from an establishment that keeps them refrigerated, and buy small quantities so your supply stays fresh.

Ginkgo Biloba. This popular ancient herbal remedy is made from a leaf extract and is thought to improve memory ability by inhibiting oxidative cell damage and improving cerebral circulation. It has been used for mild forms of age-related memory loss, early Alzheimer's disease, and other dementias. A recent systematic study review concluded that ginkgo appears to be safe, and that the evidence for memory benefits is promising, although additional studies are recommended. Initial research has found ginkgo to be helpful for treating leg cramps caused by poor circulation, a condition known as intermittent claudication. Studies of its use for the eye disease macular degeneration and for tinnitus (ringing in the ears) have been inconclusive. Possible side effects include nausea, heartburn, headaches, dizziness, excessive bruising or bleeding, and low blood pressure. Because ginkgo biloba has anticoagulant properties, taking it along with aspirin and other blood-thinning drugs requires careful monitoring.

Glucosamine and Chondroitin. Glucosamine, derived from shellfish, and chondroitin sulfate, derived from cow cartilage, are the components of a popular supplement combination used as a treatment for arthritis sufferers. Systematic studies have found that a daily combination of 1500 mg of glucosamine and 1200 mg of chondroitin sulfate not only reduces arthritis symptoms just as well as nonsteroidal anti-inflammatory drugs, but also may slow joint deterioration. The most common side effects are intestinal gas and softened stools. People with diabetes should check their blood-sugar levels more frequently when taking this supplement. The combination can interact with other medicines such as aspirin, which thin the blood. Those allergic to shellfish should consult with their doctor before taking glucosamine.

Echinacea. This herbal preparation comes from the same plant family as sunflowers and daisies. In the 1960s, it became a popular treatment for the common cold, in part because of laboratory studies suggesting that it may boost the immune system. In a recent study published in the *New England Journal of Medicine,* researchers found that echinacea was no different than a placebo in treating or preventing the symptoms of colds. Although echinacea advocates argue that the study doses were inadequate, the findings raise skepticism about whether echinacea has any effect on the common cold.

SAMe (S-adenosylmethionine). This naturally occurring compound plays a role in the immune system, maintains cell membranes, and helps produce and break down important brain chemical messengers. Research on SAMe suggests that it may be useful in the treatment of depression and arthritis. A recent study found that SAMe was as effective as traditional anti-inflammatory drugs in reducing pain and increasing mobility in patients with arthritis. Possible side effects include dry mouth, nausea, diarrhea, headache, and insomnia.

Policosanol. This supplement contains fatty alcohols derived from waxes of plants. Studies have found it to be effective in lowering the "bad" LDL cholesterol and raising levels of the "good" HDL cholesterol. Potential side effects include upset stomach, headache, and weight loss. Despite claims, no evidence supports the use of policosanol to boost energy or sexual performance.

Estrogen and Testosterone. Recent studies have left women confused about the pros and cons of taking hormone replacement therapy after menopause, and whether to take estrogen alone or estrogen plus a progestin. The Women's Health Initiative Study found that women age sixty-five and older taking different combinations of estrogen and a progestin (Premarin and Provera) had twice the likelihood of developing dementia than women who took a placebo. It is still possible that estrogen may protect the brain if taken in a different form, or earlier in life (right after menopause), but there is not yet enough evidence to recommend estrogen for dementia prevention.

Even though estrogen has not been found to prevent dementia, it does relieve menopausal symptoms. To help women make a more informed choice, the North American Menopause Society convened a panel of experts to help analyze the available research evidence and make recommendations. These experts concluded that estrogen (in pills or skin patches) should definitely be considered for younger women experiencing menopause, since estrogen helps relieve hot flashes, night sweats, and sleep disturbances caused by hot flashes. Estrogen is also an effective treatment for vaginal dryness, atrophy, or thinning, which can lead to irritation and infection. A vaginal estrogen cream, tablet, or ring is recommended for such symptoms.

Although estrogen increases the risk for uterine cancer, progestin protects against this risk. Women who have had their uterus removed don't need to take progestin when they use estrogen. Hormone therapy has been associated with increased risk for breast cancer, but more research is needed to determine the degree of risk at different ages. Hormone therapy does increase breast density, making it more difficult to detect abnormalities on mammograms, but ultrasound machines can be used, as well, to examine breasts for abnormal growths that might go undetected by mammograms in very dense breasts. Experts agree that if a woman decides to use hormone replacement therapy in order to relieve menopause symptoms, it is best to use the lowest dose she can, for the shortest amount of time. Also, her need for treatment should be reevaluated every year.

Approximately one out of five men sixty-five and older develop an abnormally low testosterone level; however, some men with normal levels augment their testosterone in an attempt to cure memory complaints, fatigue, low sex drive, and shrinking muscle mass. Although, in some cases, testosterone may improve these symptoms, it does pose risks—older men often have inactive cancer cells in their prostates, which excess testosterone could awaken.

DHEA (Dehydroepiandrosterone). Secreted by the body's adrenal gland, DHEA is a building block for estrogen and testosterone. Because DHEA declines with age, the theory is that one could extend life expectancy and avoid age-related health problems by keeping levels high. Some initial research suggests that DHEA may help treat depression in patients who do not respond well to conventional antidepressants. Its potential for protecting brain cells suggested promise for treating dementia and memory loss, but systematic studies have not backed this up. Recently, investigators found that when given to older people, DHEA can trim belly fat and help the body use insulin more effectively. The supplement does have its down side—DHEA can increase the risk of prostate cancer. Some athletes take DHEA to build strength and bulk before big events—despite its ban by organizations such as the National Football League and the International Olympic Committee.

Growth Hormone Stimulants. These natural products, also known as growth hormone "releasers," are thought to trigger the release of chemical messengers that promise to build muscle mass, trim fat, increase energy, improve sex life, boost memory, restore hair growth and color, and strengthen the immune system. Companies marketing "hormone releaser" pills say their products are a cheaper, needle-free alternative to human growth hormone injections. The active ingredient is often arginine or another amino acid that signals the pituitary gland to release or secrete growth hormone. Although growth hormone levels decline with age, it is not known whether trying to maintain the levels that exist in young persons has any benefit. For now, muscle-building athletes and others who take these products should be cautious of potential side effects, and they should know that, so far, there is minimal evidence of any benefit.

Looking Better

Remaining young-looking and attractive is an important quality longevity goal for many people. However, being comfortable in our own skin is what truly counts; and often this means aging gracefully and celebrating every well-deserved line and wrinkle. Some people choose to adamantly fight the physical signs of aging, and maintain their youthful appearance as long as possible.

When we feel that we look good, it boosts our self-esteem and confidence, which can lead to a more positive outlook, more fulfilling relationships, and other quality longevity benefits. There are a variety of approaches to looking young, ranging from face creams to surgeries.

Billions of dollars are spent every year on cosmetics to help people look younger by taking care of their skin and enhancing their appearance. Experts agree that the best way to minimize wrinkles is to avoid sun exposure, use moisturizers, and always wear sunscreen (see Essential 5). Many people, particularly women, use cosmetics to create a more youthful look (see box).

Using Makeup to Look Younger

Many people wear makeup, and experts agree it's best to apply moisturizer and sunscreen before foundation. At about middle-age and older, the face tends to take on a gray or yellowish cast, so cosmetologists advise choosing creamy foundations in beige or golden tones, and pumping up the color on the lips and cheeks — moving away from browns, and selecting more corals or rose-color tints. Avoiding powders if the skin is dry will keep the powder from settling into lines and help give the skin a dewy appearance. However, applying a soft-shade blushing powder on the cheekbones going outward and slightly upward gives definition to the face.

Grooming eyebrows gives the illusion of lifted lids, and having more skin showing at the brow bone opens up the entire eye. Using a lash curler before applying mascara also makes eyes look more open.

Thinning and graying hair can be common as we age. Many hair experts suggest either overall color to cover gray or perhaps augmenting with golden or honey highlights to add dimension, brighten the face, and make hair look thicker. As women get older, they may find it more attractive to lighten and brighten their hair color, rather than darken it.

COSMETIC MEDICINE

Each year, millions of Americans choose to undergo medical treatments or surgical techniques to improve their appearance, and make themselves look younger and healthier. Although some individuals can go too far with plastic surgery, most cosmetic-medicine consumers are simply trying to look and feel better about themselves.

When considering cosmetic surgery, a person should be clear

about his or her motivation. Pressure from friends, family, or a loved one is not the best reason to go forward. Cosmetic surgery is usually an elective procedure—something the patient *wants*, as opposed to *needs*. Also, it is important to be realistic about what any particular procedure can and cannot accomplish. Cosmetic surgery will not cure a clinical depression, although it may help you to look a lot more attractive when visiting the psychiatrist.

Choosing the right surgeon, perhaps one who specializes in the particular procedure you have chosen, is critical. A good strategy is to rely on recommendations from physicians and friends you trust. You can also check with the American Board of Plastic Surgery or the American Society of Plastic and Reconstructive Surgeons (888-475-2784 or *www.plasticsurgery.org*), although keep in mind that simply being a member of a professional society does not ensure a surgeon's quality.

Learn all you can about the procedure you will be having, and talk with the doctor about potential risks and benefits. Ask the specialist to show you photographic examples of his or her work— "before" and "after"—and be skeptical of guaranteed promises or extravagant claims.

The following section includes some of the more popular procedures that are currently available. They differ in cost, degree of invasiveness, recovery time, potential complications, and long-term outcomes, all of which should be discussed in advance with the doctor.

SURGICAL TECHNIQUES

Face Lifts. To get an idea of how your face might appear after a lift, look at yourself in a mirror while lying on your back. A face lift can smooth out wrinkles, loose skin, a sagging neck, and other aging changes. The procedure involves camouflaged incisions around the ears and usually some repositioning of the skin, as well as of the underlying tissue. A forehead or brow lift corrects drooping brows and smooths the horizontal lines and furrows that can make a person appear angry, sad, or tired. It restores a youthful, natural look to the upper third of the face. The incisions are hidden just behind the hairline.

These procedures can subtract years from someone's appearance, but there are occasional complications, including infection, bleeding, or a wide-eyed, unnatural appearance. However, in recent years, the aim has shifted toward more subtle results, rather than a drastic change in appearance, and less invasive "minilifts" have become popular. The results are less dramatic than complete face lifts, but the costs and risk of complications are lower. Minilifts and other minimally invasive procedures, such as endoscopic neck and midface lifts, are frequently used in younger patients who have reasons to justify doing a procedure, but who do not need a more comprehensive surgical intervention.

Breast Lifts. These procedures, often performed in an outpatient setting, reverse the natural sagging that occurs from age, pregnancy, breast feeding, and weight fluctuations. New techniques reduce visible scarring after the procedure, and most women are pleased with their outcome. Complications may include loss of sensation in the nipple, an unnatural appearance to the breast, and scarring.

Liposuction. This technique helps sculpt the body by removing unwanted fat from the abdomen, hips, buttocks, thighs, knees, upper arms, chin, cheeks, or neck. The surgeon injects fluid into the fat tissue and suctions out the fat along with the fluid. New methods, including ultrasound-assisted lipoplasty (UAL), the tumescent technique, and the super-wet technique, are helping plastic surgeons provide some patients with more precise results and quicker recovery times. Although it is not a substitute for dieting and exercise, liposuction can reduce stubborn areas of fat that don't respond to traditional weight-loss methods.

Liposuction, which usually requires general anesthesia, can have permanent effects if the patient is able to avoid future weight gain. Possible side effects include bleeding, infection, numbness, or a bumpy appearance to the area, if fat removal is uneven. An extremely rare and unfortunate complication is pulmonary embolism, which can cause death.

Eyelid Surgery. With age, the skin around the eyes loses elasticity and the resulting loose folds and creases can cause a puffy, tired look. Cosmetic eyelid surgery can remove the excess skin, bags, and fat from around the upper and lower eyelids. This outpatient procedure can yield long-lasting results, with patients typically appearing refreshed and rested. Complications may include eye irritation, dryness, bleeding, and loss of the natural shape of the eye from overcorrection of excess skin.

Lasik Eye Surgery. Many people who want to stop wearing glasses opt for this outpatient procedure, a relatively quick and painless way to correct vision. The surgeon makes a thin flap on the surface of the cornea, lifts the flap, and reshapes the underlying cornea with a laser. Flattening the center of the cornea corrects nearsightedness. Farsighted people have a ring of tissue around the center of the cornea removed, in order to make the cornea steeper. For people with astigmatism, the oblong-shaped cornea is made more spherical.

Although most patients get twenty-twenty vision after the procedure, those with more serious myopia, farsightedness, or astigmatism may have less than optimal results. Temporary side effects may include eye dryness, or seeing imaginary halos or spots of light. Very rarely, patients may develop infection or permanent damage to their vision.

For some patients, conductive keratoplasty, a minimally invasive procedure that does not require incisions, is effective for the treatment of mild farsightedness. It uses electrical energy to reshape the cornea. It not only allows patients to see at a distance, but can also create blended vision, so they can forgo reading glasses, as well.

Surgical Hair Enhancement. Hair transplants involve taking tiny hair follicles from the back or side of the scalp and implanting them into balding areas, typically on the crown of the head or the front of the hairline. Another technique, known as scalp reduction, involves minimizing an area of bald skin on the head by surgically removing it and stretching hair-bearing scalp in its place. Both procedures can be combined to provide a natural-appearing hair line. Rare complications of surgical hair enhancements may include infection, scarring, or further hair loss.

NONSURGICAL TREATMENTS

Botox Injections. Those crow's-feet around the eyes and frown lines on the face that accrue over the years can now be smoothed out with Botox injections. Derived from the bacteria that cause botulism, Botox literally paralyzes the muscles for a period of four to six months. The recovery time from injections is brief and improvement is usually observed within two weeks. Potential side effects include drooping upper eyelids and less facial expression due to difficulty raising the eyebrows. Recent research suggests that Botox injections may stave off migraine headaches.

Collagen Injections. Collagen is a natural protein that provides texture and soft-tissue support throughout the body. When small amounts are injected into collagen-weak areas, depressions in the surrounding skin are raised, and the area appears smoother. Although collagen injections can be effective in lessening wrinkles around the eyes, mouth, and nasolabial folds, the benefits last only a few months. A test injection, usually on the inside of the forearm, is necessary to determine if the patient is among the four percent of individuals allergic to the commonly used collagen derived from cows.

Cosmoderm and Cosmoplast, FDA-approved facial fillers, can be used without pretesting for allergic reactions. These purified human collagen treatments are bioengineered from living human cells. For lips, in particular, collagen treatment of some type is recommended as a preliminary trial before considering placement of a longer-lasting material, such as Restylane or fat injections.

Restylane Injections. Collagen has been replaced by Restylane as the most popular filler. Restylane lasts at least twice as long—up to six to nine months—and requires no pretreatment skin test. Restylane is derived from synthetic hyaluronic acid, and allergic reactions occur in less than one percent of those injected. Since 1996, over one million patients have been treated in more than sixty countries.

Fat Injections. This outpatient procedure is often performed in conjunction with liposuction and is similar to injecting collagen, but has the advantage of not producing allergic reactions. The suctioned fat from an unwanted area of the body is reinjected to smooth out wrinkled areas or to augment lips.

Mesotherapy. Cellulite is the dimpled skin that can appear on the hips, thighs, and buttocks of people as they age. Mesotherapy involves injecting medicines and other substances into the layer of fat and connective tissue under the skin, known as the mesoderm, where the cellulite is located. The procedure is still being studied, so its effectiveness is not known and it has not been accepted by the established medical community. Possible complications include infection, irregular contouring, and scarring.

Microdermabrasion. This procedure involves gently sandblasting the face, usually by spraying tiny crystals and vacuuming the resulting debris. It helps repair facial skin damaged by the sun and aging, but the benefits last for only a few months. Microdermabrasion is basically painless and requires no recovery time, but it can cause mild swelling and redness for a day.

Laser Resurfacing. This method uses high energy laser light to vaporize the outer skin layers, which then grow back smoother and tighter. Laser resurfacing can smooth out deep wrinkles and fine lines around the mouth or eyes and can last for years. Initial recovery time is usually seven to ten days, during which crusting resolves. Possible complications include loss of skin pigmentation, scarring, and sun sensitivity. Some people have pink or red skin for up to six months after the treatment, which may require concealing makeup.

Fraxel Laser. This new technique, also known as Fractional Resurfacing Technology, delivers laser light to only a fraction of the skin through a series of microscopic, closely spaced laser spots, while preserving normal healthy skin between the laser spots. This preservation of healthy skin results in rapid healing following the laser treatment. Fraxel laser can treat the entire face in approximately thirty minutes and requires three to five sessions spaced several weeks apart. It has been used effectively on the face, neck, chest, arms, and hands for photodamaged skin (brown spots), fine and moderate wrinkles, and acne scarring. The procedure involves minimal discomfort and causes only slight redness for a day or two, followed by bronzing of the skin for about a week.

Radio Wave Therapy. The FDA recently approved radio wave therapy as a nonsurgical treatment for wrinkles. The technique, sometimes marketed as Thermage, involves a spray that cools the skin surface while radio waves are emitted and penetrate to deeper skin layers, particularly the collagen layer. There is some immediate tightening of the collagen fibers, which smooths the overlying skin. Eventually, new collagen grows from the heat stimulus of the radio waves, which further tightens the skin over a two- to six-month period.

Photofacial. Intense Pulsed Light Therapy, or IPL, can eliminate dark aging spots, sun freckles, and superficial capillaries, as well as diminish fine wrinkles and tighten pores in the skin. This form of photorejuvenation can be utilized as a treatment for rosacea, or simply to improve the tone and texture of the skin. It is FDA approved and usually requires four to six treatments. Patients looking to revitalize their appearance without any down time often choose this procedure.

Chemical Peels. This method improves the appearance of the skin on the face, neck, chest, and hands. A chemical solution is applied to the skin, causing it to peel off so that new, smoother, regenerated skin replaces the older, wrinkled skin. Chemical peels can improve fine lines under the eyes and around the mouth, mild scarring, and acne, as well as wrinkles from sun damage and aging. However, deeper wrinkles generally do not respond unless the clinician uses a more concentrated acid solution, which may result in skin or pigment loss and an unnatural change in skin texture. After a peel, the new skin is temporarily more sensitive to the sun. Superficial peels usually result in redness, followed by scaling for up to a week. Deeper peels may lead to swelling, blisters, and crusting for up to two weeks.

Skin Creams. The FDA regulates the safety of many skin-care products, but doesn't really concern itself with their effectiveness. Product brand names can often be deceptive, sometimes alluding to cosmetic surgery–like results—for example, the "mini-lift miracle cream" or the "botoxin-smoothie mask." Many of the latest products contain a small fragment of protein that is absorbed into the skin's top layer. These fragments are thought to stimulate collagen production, which smooths the skin. Some creams actually contain collagen, but these tend to be less effective, because collagen has to be injected in order for it to penetrate the skin. Other ingredients in many products, including actual DNA molecules or hyaluronic acid, have not been demonstrated to show benefits. These creams *do* help to moisturize the skin, which any effective skin cream or lotion can do.

Another cream ingredient is a vitamin A derivative (e.g., Retin-A or Renova), which can tighten the skin and replace old skin with new skin. Noticeable improvement may take months, and potential side effects include temporary redness, scaling, burning, itching, and thinning of the skin over time.

Medicines for Hair Growth. Although baldness has become a cool look for some men, many still define their youthful self-image by how much hair they have on their head. Some women also experience hair loss as they get older. Two drugs are available for the treatment of balding: minoxidil, marketed as Rogaine, and finasteride, marketed as Propecia or Proscar. Both medicines help stave off future hair loss, and can sometimes stimulate the growth of new hair.

Rogaine is rubbed onto the scalp twice daily—the new hair may be thinner and shorter than previous hair, but it can blend in and help hide bald spots. It occasionally causes scalp irritation. Propecia is a prescription pill that is taken once daily and usually shows results within a few months. Rarely, it can decrease sex drive, and as with Rogaine, the benefits stop if the medicine is discontinued.

Keeping Your Smile Young. As we get older, our gums tend to recede, which exposes some of the roots of our teeth, making them more susceptible to infection and decay. Gum or periodontal disease becomes more common with age, afflicting approximately 50 percent of people fifty-five years and older. In addition to decay, it can cause tooth loss and bleeding, which allows bacteria to enter the bloodstream and contribute to inflammation throughout the body. This may be why gum disease increases the risk of heart disease or stroke. A recent study also found that gum disease early in life increases the risk for Alzheimer's disease late in life.

Although genetics plays a role in the risk for gum disease, proper brushing and flossing are the best defense, and can even offset a genetic risk. When brushing, use a brush with small and soft bristles. To help reduce decay, brush with a fluoride toothpaste and floss at least twice daily. Ask your dentist or dental hygienist to review your technique, and be sure to get your teeth cleaned at regular intervals. Avoid mouth dryness by taking small sips of water throughout the day. Also, brush or rinse after eating sweet or sticky foods such as raisins. A cosmetic dentist can also advise you on procedures to improve the appearance of your smile and teeth, such as whitening products and bonding.

Staying Young with Modern Medicine

- Medical breakthroughs are focusing on early detection and prevention of disease before damage sets in. Becoming informed consumers of new medical technologies and treatments helps us live longer, and look and feel younger.
- Don't hesitate to get help—screen early rather than late for illnesses such as osteoporosis, cancer, diabetes, and hypertension.
- Augment your medicine's benefits by exercising, eating right, eliminating stress, and embracing the other quality longevity essentials.
- Listen to your doctor's advice—taking the correct medicine in the right way can add healthy years to your life. Don't use more medicines than you need, and discuss side effects with your doctor.
- Libido boosters and sexual enhancers for both men and women can help keep sex a vital part of life, well into old age.
- If you decide on a cosmetic treatment or procedure, make sure to review the pros and cons of the many options available.

Part 3

Putting It All Together

The secret of longevity is to keep breathing.

—SOPHIE TUCKER

People start getting proactive about their quality longevity at various stages of life, and for many different reasons. Some are like Nancy G., whose family history of Alzheimer's disease motivated her to take charge. Or Shirley I., whose memory slips encouraged her to get involved. Sometimes all it takes to motivate someone to pursue a *Longevity Bible* lifestyle is a little age reminder such as a new line in your face, or perhaps noticing how much older people look at your high school reunion.

Regardless of your reason for pursuing a longer, healthier, and more youthful life, you now have some knowledge of the Eight Essential areas where you *do* have some control. How much you need to emphasize each area will depend on your current strengths and needs, as well as the feasibility of making changes that fit in with your lifestyle. If your job involves a lot of travel, adhering to the Longevity Diet will be a challenge, but it is definitely achievable. If you are a long-distance runner, you probably don't need to worry about upgrading your level of physical activity. If you happen to be a rocket scientist, you may not need to spend too much time doing mental aerobics. This means you will have more time to concentrate on the other essential areas.

Working the Eight Essentials Together

When we work several of the Eight Essentials together, we benefit from the synergy of their combined effects. Your particular quality longevity challenges will determine the specifics of your *Longevity Bible* program, and the program itself will continually change as you achieve results in one area and then find yourself able to focus more on another area. Eating a healthy longevity diet as well as sharpening your mind can lead to a more positive attitude. This often benefits your relationships and may lead you to experience less stress in your life. As a result, you may be able to cut back on your relationship exercises and the amount of time you spend each day on stress reduction. This in turn can free up more time for improving your environment by decluttering some of the rooms in your apartment or house. You may also have more time to work out, which can help lower your blood pressure and reduce the need for medicines.

To help you individualize your quality longevity program, first review the following key points for achieving each of the Eight Essentials. Place a check mark next to the points you feel you need to emphasize as you begin your program. Then review the details of those essentials to fine-tune the strategies you've chosen.

Sharpen Your Mind

Regular mental activity will help keep the mind sharp, improve memory skills, and protect the brain from future decline. When combined with the other *Longevity Bible* Essential Strategies, it not

☐ To get the most out of your mental workouts, apply the *P*'s and *Q*'s for Sharpening the Mind: 1) maintain *presence* and focus; 2) *persevere* in your endeavors to further sharpen your mind; 3) look for the *quality* and meaning in things; and 4) always *question* to learn more.

☐ Try different approaches to expanding your mental horizons, such as traveling to new destinations, learning a musical instrument, taking up ballroom dancing, or going back to school.

☐ Learn and practice the three basic memory techniques:

–Look: Focus attention on what you want to remember

–Snap: Imagine a mental snapshot of the information

–Connect: Link the snapshots together in your mind's eye

☐ Practice more advanced memory strategies for remembering names and faces.

☐ Stay mentally active through puzzles, games, reading, and other stimulating hobbies, but be sure to train and not strain your brain—find the level of mental challenge that keeps you interested without frustrating or exhausting you.

only makes people feel happier and function more effectively, but it may also extend life expectancy.

Keep a Positive Outlook

A positive outlook helps us live longer and stay healthier. Optimists have fewer physical and emotional difficulties, experience less pain, enjoy higher energy levels, and are generally happier and calmer in their lives. Although genetics plays a role, scientific evi-

☐ Make a conscious effort to be extroverted and energetic—happiness is contagious.

☐ Forgive yourself and others who wrong you—letting go of grudges lowers stress levels and fosters a positive outlook.

☐ Build self-esteem by making moral choices. Keep in mind your accomplishments and successes to help rebut your inner self-critic.

☐ If you don't already have an active spiritual or religious life, consider getting involved in one, whether it's through meditation, organized religion, seeking harmony with nature, or any other method.

☐ Learn to be optimistic through simple, systematic approaches. Recognize what your negativity triggers are, and challenge any negative assumptions you are quick to make.

☐ Avoid pessimistic thinking by focusing on your strengths and setting achievable and realistic goals.

☐ Don't be a loner—ask others for support and get professional help if you need it.

dence shows that maintaining a positive attitude, like any other skill, can be learned.

Cultivate Healthy and Intimate Relationships

Staying socially connected not only bolsters physical and emotional well-being, it reduces stress levels and can add years to our lives. Empathy and other basic skills that help us stay connected to others can be learned and improved upon, and even the most social among us can fine-tune his or her skills.

☐ Stay connected and involved socially, whether you are single or in a couple. Try to spend time with a healthy crowd.

☐ Reduce relationship clutter by cutting loose unsatisfying or "toxic" friends and acquaintances.

☐ Develop and maintain your empathy skills. Listen to others, try to identify with their feelings, and let them know that you understand.

☐ If you are in an intimate relationship, make efforts to nurture it: Schedule time together, share feelings without criticizing, and stay in touch with friends and other couples. A healthy sex life adds to quality longevity.

☐ Having a pet may contribute to longer life expectancy. Pets can also be enjoyable, stress-reducing companions.

☐ Planning ahead for the emotional and practical challenges of parent care can make the role-reversal much less stressful for both older parents and their adult children, should the need arise.

Promote Stress-Free Living

Chronic stress has been associated with an increased risk for cancer, high blood pressure, and heart disease, and may speed up the very aging of our cells by a decade or more. Stress impairs memory, and makes us look and feel older. Although we cannot control all of the outside factors that contribute to stress in our lives, we *can* have a major impact on how we react to stress, and minimize its influence on our health and longevity.

- ☐ Practice mindful awareness—staying in the moment and being aware of what is going on inside your body—through meditation, relaxation techniques, yoga, or other exercises you enjoy. Take stress release breaks throughout the day.
- ☐ Avoid multitasking by scheduling a regular time each day for completing priority chores; try finishing one task before beginning another.
- ☐ Learn to say "no" when you need to.
- ☐ Modulate stress with healthy expressions of anger.
- ☐ Use humor to gain perspective on stressful situations.
- ☐ Get a good night's sleep every night. Take simple steps to beat insomnia without medication.
- ☐ Discover ways to limit stress on the job.
- ☐ Place emphasis on saving for the future.
- ☐ Reduce stress by decluttering your personal environment.
- ☐ Plan your strategy for dealing with stressful events you know about in advance.

Master Your Environment

Our environment has a major influence on how we feel and how long we live. Whether it's traffic, noise, smog, or other aspects of the environment at large, or more personal environmental issues such as clutter, aesthetics, or bedroom temperature, our quality longevity requires that we not only adapt to these influences, but learn to shape them to meet our individual tastes and needs. Consider the following personal solutions for environmental issues, and check off any that could be helpful for your longevity program.

☐ Bear in mind function and aesthetics when designing your home and work space. Control clutter and noise, and arrange the bedroom in a way that enhances sleep and restfulness.

☐ Minimize your exposure to sun, smoke, mold, smog, and other airborne toxins.

☐ Stay safe on the road—let someone else drive if you can't handle it.

☐ Make your workplace safe and comfortable: Consider ergonomic designs for comfort and safety.

☐ Manage your technology to avoid information overload.

☐ If parent care becomes a reality, consider the advantages and disadvantages of various housing choices.

☐ Help conserve natural resources and protect your environment.

Body Fitness—Shape Up to Stay Young

Physical activity, whether it's walking, cycling, playing tennis, or dancing, keeps us living longer, feeling healthier, and looking younger. Even a short, brisk ten-minute daily walk can reduce the risk of age-related diseases such as Alzheimer's. Physically active people also have lower rates of heart attacks, cancer, diabetes, and depression, and these benefits can be experienced at almost any age. The Longevity Fitness Routine promotes health and boosts energy levels.

- ☐ Sample different types of cardiovascular exercise methods and choose one or more that you find fun and challenging. Sports and exercise protect your body *and* your mind.
- ☐ Exercise with a friend—getting physical *and* social reduces stress and keeps you connected to others.
- ☐ Divide your routine among the three vital Longevity Fitness areas:
  –Cardiovascular conditioning
  –Balance and flexibility
  –Strength training
- ☐ Exercise several days a week—don't be a weekend warrior.
- ☐ Build strength and stamina gradually to maximize fitness and avoid injury—push yourself to the next level only when you're ready.
- ☐ If you have an ongoing medical condition, be sure to check with your doctor before starting any exercise program.

The Longevity Diet

Diet directly impacts our health and life expectancy by affecting our risk for heart disease, cancer, and other age-related illnesses. It also influences our appearance and mental state. The Longevity Diet is based on the latest scientific evidence on foods that improve health and lengthen life, and it still allows us to occasionally get away with eating our favorite cheat eats without guilt. Learning to "cross-train" our eating among healthy food groups allows us to break free of the boredom and repetition of many of today's popular diets.

☐ Eat the foods you like the most from the following food groups every day. Each food group can *star* in up to two meals per day.
  –Antioxidant fruits and vegetables
  –Proteins, lean meats, and healthy fats
  –Whole grains, legumes, and other carbohydrates
☐ Use mindful awareness to focus on how your body feels before, during, and after eating, to help you gauge portion size and know when you've had enough.
☐ Occasionally indulge in a small portion of your favorite cheat eats.
☐ Drink at least eight glasses of water throughout the day.
☐ Enjoy two to three healthy between-meal snacks a day.
☐ Avoid excessive salts, bad fats, and high-glycemic carbohydrates.
☐ If you wish to lose weight, cut back on carbohydrates, alcohol, and cheat eats until you reach your goal.

Modern Medicine for Feeling and Looking Younger

Today's medical technology is keeping our generation living longer, as well as looking and feeling better than any generation before us. By combining a healthy lifestyle with new disease-detection methods, better medicines and vaccines, and novel surgical procedures, we can expect a significant increase in the number of years we live, as well as the health and youthfulness we enjoy during

- ☐ Medical breakthroughs are focusing on early detection and prevention of disease before damage sets in. Becoming informed consumers of new medical technologies and treatments helps us to live longer, and look and feel younger.
- ☐ Don't hesitate to get help—screen early rather than late for illnesses such as osteoporosis, cancer, diabetes, and hypertension.
- ☐ Augment your medicine's benefits by exercising, eating right, eliminating stress, and embracing the other quality longevity essentials.
- ☐ Listen to your doctor's advice—taking the correct medicine in the right way can add healthy years to your life. Don't use more medicines than you need, and discuss side effects with your doctor.
- ☐ Libido boosters and sexual enhancers for both men and women can help keep sex a vital part of life, well into old age.
- ☐ If you decide on a cosmetic treatment or procedure, make sure to review the pros and cons of the many options available.

those years. With the range of treatments and procedures now available, it is essential to become an informed consumer, choosing and monitoring our own *medical portfolios* wisely.

Getting With the Program

When beginning a *Longevity Bible* Program, many people find it helpful to set short-term and long-term goals for each of the Eight Essentials. After reviewing the checklists, Alan F. came up with the following list of goals:

GOALS

8 Essentials	Short-Term	Long-Term
Sharp Mind	1. Start doing daily crossword puzzles. 2. Take guitar lessons.	Lower risk for Alzheimer's.
Attitude	1. Inner-critic exercises twice this week. 2. Start going to church on Sundays.	Increase self- confidence.
Relationships	1. Try attentive-listening exercises. 2. Go away with girlfriend on weekend.	Eventually get married; feel closer to kids.
Stress-Free	1. Go to yoga classes. 2. Delegate tasks to reduce workload.	Feel less anxious.
Environment	1. Wear sunscreen. 2. Have mildew-smelling basement checked for toxic mold.	Reduce risk for cancer and other illnesses.
Body Fitness	1. Take a 10-minute walk after dinner. 2. Begin Longevity Fitness Routine.	Increase stamina; avoid injuries.
Diet	1. Cut back on red meat and salt. 2. Get more whole grains into diet.	Lose ten pounds and lower blood pressure.
Medicine	1. Take daily blood pressure medicine. 2. Get colonoscopy this month.	Lower blood pressure and detect treatable illnesses.

The synergy of the Eight Essentials helped Alan F. make quick gains in his quality longevity. With his increased confidence, he became less defensive and more comfortable about moving forward in his relationship with his girlfriend. He also started feeling closer to his son. The stress reduction from his yoga classes lowered his anxiety levels. This, along with his low-salt diet, made it possible for his doctor to reduce his blood pressure medicine. When Alan became more proactive by delegating some of his work tasks, he had more leisure time, which lowered his stress levels further and allowed him to spend more time with the people he cared about in his life.

Alan tried not to obsess over every detail of his longevity program. Within each of the Eight Essentials, he didn't focus on everything all at once, but started on the areas in which he felt he could use the most work. This allowed him to enjoy the benefits of his efforts as soon as possible. Once a person begins to achieve his or her short-term goals, that individual usually gains motivation to take on even greater challenges, which can further increase the quality and number of his or her years ahead.

In the Appendices that follow, you'll find additional resources for more help with the Eight Essentials. I've included some recipes you may want to try as you become familiar with the Longevity Diet, as well as more mental aerobics exercises to use for additional brain workouts.

None of us will live forever, but we *can* take greater control of how well and how long we live. Our genes don't have the final word on our quality longevity trajectory. Starting a *Longevity Bible* lifestyle today will help you live to enjoy the benefits for years to come.

Appendix 1

The Longevity Diet Recipes

APPLE CRUMBLE À LA MODE

(makes 4–6 servings)

4 apples, peeled and thinly sliced
¼ teaspoon cinnamon
⅔ cup whole-grain and oat granola
2 cups frozen vanilla yogurt or fat-free vanilla ice cream

Preheat the oven to 350°F. Lightly coat a small baking dish with cooking spray and arrange the apples in the dish. Sprinkle them with the cinnamon and granola. Bake until the fruit is bubbling, about 30 minutes. Let cool 5 to 10 minutes. Scoop the frozen yogurt into bowls and top with baked apple crumble. Serve immediately.

Variation: Can also be prepared with berries, nectarines, peaches, pears, or plums.

BUTTERMILK DRESSING, LOWFAT

(makes 2 cups)

1 cup nonfat sour cream
1 cup reduced-fat buttermilk
2 tablespoons honey
2 tablespoons scallions, minced
Kosher salt and freshly cracked black pepper, to taste

In a small bowl, whisk together the sour cream, buttermilk, and honey. Fold in the scallions and season with salt and pepper.

CARAMELIZED ONION DIP

1 tablespoon extra-virgin olive oil
½ sweet onion, finely chopped
1 tablespoon balsamic vinegar
1 cup nonfat sour cream
1 teaspoon garlic powder
1 teaspoon seasoning salt
Fresh sliced vegetables for dipping

Heat the olive oil and onion in a nonstick skillet, over medium heat. Sauté the onions until they begin to soften and caramelize, stirring occasionally, about 15 minutes. Add the balsamic vinegar and continue to sauté until balsamic vinegar is nearly dry. Allow the onion to cool completely and fold into the sour cream. Add the garlic powder and seasoning salt, and mix well. Refrigerate for at least 30 minutes before serving. Serve with sliced vegetables for dipping.

CHEESY PESTO WITH PASTA

(makes 6–8 side servings)

1   package frozen chopped spinach, thawed and drained
4   cloves garlic, crushed
⅔ cup lowfat cottage cheese
⅔ cup fresh basil, chopped (or substitute 4 tablespoons dried)
½ cup parmesan cheese, grated
½ cup pine nuts
2   tablespoons olive oil
⅔ cup hot water
8   ounces whole-grain pasta (fusilli, spaghetti, or linguini)

In a food processor or blender, mix the spinach, garlic, cottage cheese, and basil. Separate a small amount of the parmesan cheese and pine nuts to sprinkle on top later, then add the rest to the mixture, along with the olive oil and water. Process until smooth, adding more water if needed. Toss warm pasta with desired amount of pesto sauce, and top with remaining parmesan cheese and pine nuts. Store leftover pesto in refrigerator or freezer.

FIVE-MINUTE FAT-FREE CHILLED STRAWBERRY SOUP

(makes 4 servings)

1   quart fresh strawberries, stems removed
12   ounces fat-free vanilla yogurt
A pinch or two of ground ginger
Juice of 1 orange
4–6 fresh mint leaves

Place ingredients in food processor or blender and puree until smooth. Chill and serve with a small dollop of yogurt and a mint sprig as garnish.

FENNEL, ORANGE, AND RED ONION SALAD

(makes 4 servings)

2 large bulbs fennel, quartered and cored
1 bag designer baby arugula
½ red onion, thinly sliced
1 can unsweetened mandarin oranges
2–3 tablespoons extra-virgin olive oil
Salt and pepper, to taste

Thinly slice the fennel and place in a large bowl with the arugula and red onion. Drain the juice from the mandarin oranges into a small bowl, and add the orange sections to the fennel and arugula. Whisk the olive oil into the reserved orange juice and season with salt and pepper. Toss the dressing with the salad.

GREEN BEANS WITH LEMON

(makes 4 servings)

1 pound fresh green beans, cleaned and trimmed
2 teaspoons fresh lemon juice
2 teaspoons finely chopped fresh flat-leaf parsley leaves
1 teaspoon freshly grated lemon zest
Salt and pepper, to taste

In a large saucepan of boiling salted water, cook beans until crisp-tender, about 3 to 4 minutes. Drain, then toss beans in a large bowl with lemon juice, parsley, and lemon zest. Season with salt and pepper.

MIXED SEAFOOD AND LINGUINI

(makes 4–6 servings)

8 ounces whole-wheat linguini
1 yellow pepper, cut into ½-inch pieces
½ cup onion, chopped
2 cloves garlic, crushed
½ teaspoon instant chicken bouillon powder
1 teaspoon dried basil
½ teaspoon dried oregano
2 tablespoons cornstarch
8 ounces scallops and 8 ounces shrimp (shelled)
2 large tomatoes, seeded and chopped
2 tablespoons fresh parsley, chopped
   Freshly grated parmesan cheese
   Freshly grated pepper, to taste

Cook the linguini and keep warm. In a large skillet, cook the yellow pepper, onion, garlic, bouillon, basil, and oregano, slowly adding one cup of water. Continue cooking until vegetables are tender, about 5 minutes. In a separate bowl, stir together the cornstarch and 2 tablespoons water, then add to vegetables. Cook until bubbling. Add shrimp and scallops and cook 3 to 4 minutes until seafood is done. Stir in tomatoes. Toss with linguini and sprinkle with parsley. Serve with grated parmesan cheese and pepper.

RAISIN-BRAN MUFFINS

(makes 12 muffins)

1 cup whole-bran cereal
1 cup nonfat milk
1 egg, slightly beaten
¼ cup canola oil
¼ cup sugar
½ teaspoon shredded lemon peel
¾ cup whole-wheat flour
¾ cup all-purpose flour
¼ teaspoon salt
2 teaspoons baking powder
¾ cup raisins

Preheat oven to 400°F. Combine cereal and milk and let moisten. Add egg, oil, sugar, and lemon peel. In a separate mixing bowl, stir flours, salt, and baking powder. Add cereal mixture to flour bowl, then stir raisins into batter. Spray a 12-cup muffin pan with nonstick cooking spray and fill each cup ⅔ full with batter. Bake 17 to 20 minutes, or until golden brown.

ROQUEFORT DRESSING

2 ounces Roquefort or blue cheese, crumbled
1 cup buttermilk (reduced fat)
¾ teaspoon sherry vinegar
½ teaspoon walnut oil
  Ground pepper to taste

In a food processor or blender, combine the cheese, buttermilk, vinegar, and oil. Process until smooth and creamy (about 1 minute), then transfer to a container and add pepper. Keeps in refrigerator up to 1 week.

SPLIT PEA SOUP, LOWFAT

(makes 8 servings)

2 quarts low-sodium chicken or vegetable stock
2 cups dried split peas
1 cup chopped celery
1 finely chopped medium onion
1 bay leaf
10 sprigs fresh flat-leaf parsley
1 medium carrot, quartered
4 slices uncooked turkey bacon

In a large stockpot combine the chicken stock, peas, celery, onion, bay leaf, parsley, carrot, and uncooked turkey bacon. Bring to a boil, reduce heat, and simmer for 1 hour. Remove and discard the bay leaf and the turkey bacon. Reserve one cup of peas. In batches, process the soup in a blender until smooth. Add the reserved peas and serve immediately.

STRAWBERRY SORBET

(makes 4–6 servings)

2 pints fresh strawberries, hulled
1½ tablespoons honey
1 teaspoon orange liqueur (optional)

Freeze the strawberries on a cookie sheet, until solid. Put in food processor and process until the texture of cornmeal. Add honey and optional liqueur and process until firm. Serve immediately or transfer to a bowl and freeze for 1 day before serving.

Variation: Sorbet can also be made with peaches or pears: Cut fruit into chunks, then toss with 1 tablespoon lemon juice before freezing. Skip the liqueur.

WHITE BEAN SALAD

16 ounces Great Northern beans
½ red bell pepper, diced
¼ cup scallions, thinly sliced
1 can white albacore tuna, drained (optional)
½ cup flat-leaf parsley, roughly chopped
1 tablespoon extra-virgin olive oil
  Juice of 1 lemon

Toss all ingredients together in a large bowl. Season with salt and pepper, to taste.

Appendix 2

More Mental Aerobics
to Tease Your Brain

1. With your nondominant hand (i.e., your left hand if you are right-handed), draw a simple three-dimensional cube. Start with a small square, then draw three diagonal lines and connect them like the figure on the right. Shade in the far side of it.

2. All of the vowels have been removed from the following proverb, and the remaining consonants are in the correct sequence broken up into groups of two to five letters. Replace the vowels and find the proverb:

FR   NDNN   DSF   RN   DNDD

3. Try to figure out the implied phrase below.

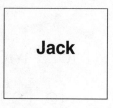

Jack

4. See how many words you can spell from the letters below. No letter may be used twice, and each word must have the letter "H" in it.

| H | S | E | R | C | A | O |

5. Starting with NOOK, change one letter at a time until you have the word BARN. Each change must be a proper word.

NOOK

. . . .

. . . .

. . . .

BARN

6. Can you make the names of three U.S. capitals from the letters below? No letter may be used more than once.

PCKOXLN   **ASHV**   **INSNI**   **EJLEHAO**

7. Which of the following words is the odd one out?

ELBAT   **AFOS**   **PMAL**   **LLAW**   **RESSERD**

8. When he has leisure time, Jim will read only certain kinds of material. He'll read *biographies*, but not *science fiction*. He likes the *sports page*, but not the *business section*. He'll review a *law journal*, but not a *mystery*. Based on this reading pattern, would he choose to read a *movie poster* or a *magazine*?

9. Figure out the missing number from the center square.

3	4	6
3		3
5	3	2

10. Mini-Crossword:

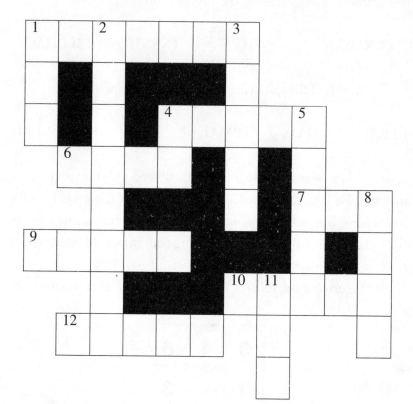

Clues

ACROSS

1. Social glue
4. Inactive potato
6. Brain teasers sharpen it
7. Cash source (abbrev.)
9. Omega-3 oil
10. Relating to birth
12. In need of relaxation

DOWN

1. Lasik target
2. Quality longevity outlook
3. *The ____ and the Restless*
4. ____ -ROM
5. Blood pumper
8. Calcium booster
11. Visually creative work

11. Which of three numbered symbols below will complete the sequence?

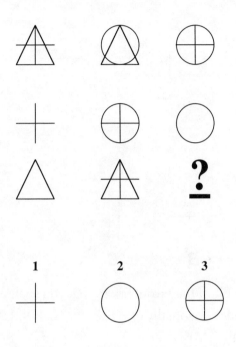

12. Figure out the message in the box below.

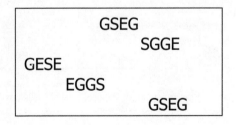

13. Which of three lettered symbols below will complete the sequence?

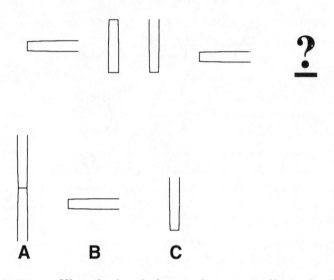

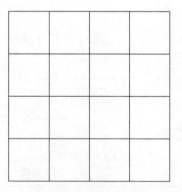

A   **B**   **C**

14. Try to fill in the box below so that you spell out the following words, either horizontally or vertically: AMEN, ENDS, LEND, MATE, MOLE, OMEN, TEND

Answers to More Mental Aerobics

1. No correct answer.
2. A friend in need is a friend indeed.

3. Jack in the box.

4. I came up with the following words:
ARCH, ARCHES, ASH, CASH, CHASE, CHORE(S), CHOSE, HARE(S), HAS, HE, HEAR(S), HO, HOE(S), HOSE, OH, RAH, RASH, SEARCH, SHARE, SHE, SHOE, SHEAR

5. NOOK, NOON, BOON, BORN, BARN

6. Phoenix, Jackson, Nashville

7. **LLAW**—All the others are pieces of furniture spelled backward.

8. A *magazine*. Jim reads only material that has the letter "a" in it.

9. 4—Each column adds up to the number 11.

10. Mini-crossword answers:

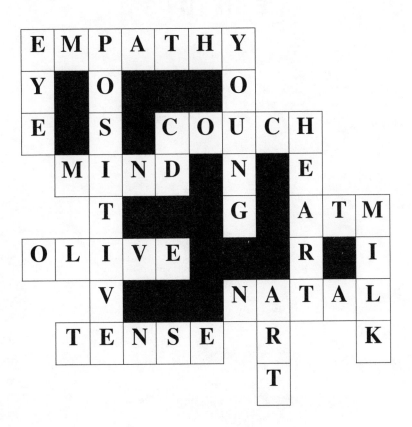

11. 1—The last symbol in each column and row is always the same as the preceding two symbols minus any part that has been duplicated.

12. SCRAMBLED EGGS

13. A—This will spell the word "couch."

14.

M	O	L	E
A	M	E	N
T	E	N	D
E	N	D	S

Appendix 3

Additional Resources

Many organizations provide information on general health and other issues important to achieving quality longevity. Several national organizations also have local or state chapters. Check your telephone directory or Internet search engine for related organizations and Web sites.

Name & Address	Description	Telephone
AARP 6601 E Street NW Washington, DC 20049 *www.aarp.org*	Nonprofit, nonpartisan organization dedicated to helping older Americans achieve lives of independence, dignity, and purpose.	888-687-2277
Academy of Molecular Imaging Box 951735 Los Angeles, CA 90095-1735 *www.ami-imaging.org*	Provides leadership in research and clinical aspects of molecular imaging of the biological nature of disease. Their Web site includes a listing of local PET centers.	310-267-2614

Name & Address	Description	Telephone
Administration on Aging Washington, DC 20201 *www.aoa.gov*	Provides information for older Americans and their families on opportunities and services to enrich their lives and support their independence.	202-619-0724
Aging Network Services 4400 East-West Highway, Suite 907 Bethesda, MD 20814 *www.agingnets.com*	Nationwide network of private-practice geriatric social workers serving as care managers for seniors living at a distance from their families.	301-657-4329
Alliance of Information and Referral Systems 11240 Waples Mill Road Suite 200 Fairfax, VA 22030 *www.airs.org*	Professional organization that provides human services information and referrals.	703-218-AIRS (2477)
Alzheimer Europe 145 Route de Thionville L-2611 Luxembourg *www.alzheimer-europe.org*	Organizes support for caregivers and raises awareness about dementia through cooperation among European Alzheimer's organizations.	352-29-79-70
Alzheimer's Association 225 N. Michigan Ave., Floor 17 Chicago, IL 60601 *www.alz.org*	National organization that provides information on Alzheimer's services, programs, publications, and local chapters.	800-272-3900

Name & Address	Description	Telephone
Alzheimer's Disease Education & Referral Center P.O. Box 8250 Silver Springs, MD 20907-8250 *www.alzheimers.org*	National Institute on Aging service that distributes information and free materials on topics relevant to health professionals, patients and their families, and the general public.	800-438-4380
Alzheimer's Foundation of America 322 Eighth Avenue, 6th floor New York, NY 10001 *www.alzfdn.org*	National nonprofit foundation supporting organizations that help lighten the burden and improve the quality of life of Alzheimer's patients and their caregivers.	866-AFA-8484 (866-232-8484)
American Academy of Neurology 1080 Montreal Avenue St. Paul, MN 55116 *www.aan.com*	Professional organization that advances the art and science of neurology, thereby promoting the best possible care for patients with neurological disorders.	651-695-2717 800-879-1960
American Association for Geriatric Psychiatry 7910 Woodmont Avenue, Suite 1050 Bethesda, MD 20814-3004 *www.aagpgpa.org*	Professional organization dedicated to enhancing the mental health and well-being of older adults, through education and research.	301-654-7850

Name & Address	Description	Telephone
American Diabetes Association Attn: National Call Center 1701 North Beauregard Street Alexandria, VA 22311 *www.diabetes.org*	America's leading nonprofit health organization, providing diabetes research, information, and advocacy.	1-800-DIABETES (800-342-2383)
American Dietetic Association 120 South Riverside Plaza, Suite 2000 Chicago, IL 60606-6995 *www.eatright.org*	Consumer nutrition hotline that provides information on finding a dietitian.	800-877-1600
American Geriatrics Society The Empire State Building 350 Fifth Avenue, Suite 801 New York, NY 10118 *www.americangeriatrics.org*	Professional association providing assistance in identifying local geriatric physician referrals.	212-308-1414
American Heart Association 7272 Greenville Avenue Dallas, TX 75231 *www.americanheart.org*	Nonprofit health organization whose mission is to reduce disability and death from cardiovascular diseases and stroke.	800-242-8721
American Psychiatric Association 1000 Wilson Blvd., Suite 1825 Arlington, VA 22209 *www.psych.org*	Medical specialty society that works to ensure humane care and effective treatment for all people with mental disorders.	888-357-7924

Name & Address	Description	Telephone
American Psychological Association 750 First Street, NE Washington, DC 20002 www.apa.org	Scientific and professional organization that represents psychology in the U.S. and aims to promote health, education, and human welfare.	800-374-2721
American Society on Aging 833 Market Street, Suite 511 San Francisco, CA 94103 www.asaging.org	National organization concerned with physical, emotional, social, economic, and spiritual aspects of aging.	415-974-9600 800-537-9728
Children of Aging Parents 1609 Woodbourne Rd., #302-A Levittown, PA 19057 www.caps4caregivers.org	National organization providing information and referrals for caregivers of older adults.	215-945-6900 800-227-7294
Dana Alliance for Brain Initiatives 745 Fifth Avenue, Suite 900 New York, NY 10151 www.dana.org	Nonprofit organization committed to advancing public awareness about the progress and benefits of brain research.	
Family Caregiver Alliance 180 Montgomery Street, Suite 1100 San Francisco, CA 94104 www.caregiver.org	Resource center for families of adults with brain damage or dementia, which provides publications for caregivers and professionals.	415-434-3388 800-445-8106

Name & Address	Description	Telephone
Gerontological Society of America 1030 15th Street NW, Suite 250 Washington, DC 20005 *www.geron.org*	National interdisciplinary organization on research and education in aging.	202-842-1275
Memory Fitness Institute 638 Camino De Los Mares, Suite H130 San Clemente, CA 92673 *www.memoryfitness institute.org*	Helps people of all ages to optimize their memory function and brain health, using state-of-the-art diagnostic, intervention, and prevention strategies.	(888) MEMFIT4
National Association of Area Agencies on Aging 1730 Rhode Island Avenue, NW, Suite 1200 Washington, DC 20036 *www.n4a.org*	Umbrella organization for the 655 area agencies on aging. Helps older people and people with disabilities live with dignity and choices in their homes and communities for as long as possible.	202-872-0888
National Center for Complementary and Alternative Medicine, National Institutes of Health 9000 Rockville Pike Bethesda, MD 20829 *www.nccam.nih.gov*	Branch of the National Institutes of Health dedicated to exploring complementary and alternative healing practices in the context of rigorous science.	888-644-6226

Name & Address	Description	Telephone
National Consumer Law Center 77 Summer Street, 10th floor Boston, MA 02110 *www.consumerlaw.org*	Nonprofit legal resource organization committed to making consumer law work for the interests of older adults and low-income individuals.	
The National Council on the Aging 300 D Street, SW, Suite 801 Washington, DC 20024 *www.ncoa.org*	National network of organizations and individuals dedicated to improving the health and independence of older persons and increasing their continuing contributions to communities, society, and future generations.	202-479-1200
National Institute of Mental Health, Public Information and Communications Branch 6001 Executive Boulevard, Room 8184, MSC 9663 Bethesda, MD 20892-9663 *www.nimh.nih.gov*	Part of the National Institutes of Health. Principal biomedical and behavioral research agency of the United States government.	866-615-6464
National Institute of Neurological Disorders and Stroke P.O. Box 5801 Bethesda, MD 20824 *www.ninds.nih.gov*	National Institutes of Health agency that supports neuroscience research. Focuses on rapidly translating scientific discoveries into prevention, treatment, and cures, and provides resource support and information.	301-496-5751 800-352-9424

Name & Address	Description	Telephone
National Institute on Aging Building 31, Room 5C27 31 Center Drive, MSC 2292 Bethesda, MD 20892 *www.nih.gov.nia*	National Institutes of Health agency that supports research on aging and provides information about national Alzheimer's centers, and a free directory of organizations that serve older adults.	301-496-1752
National Osteoporosis Foundation 1232 22nd Street, NW Washington, DC 20037-1292 *www.nof.org*	Nonprofit organization dedicated to preventing and curing osteoporosis. Supports numerous programs of awareness, education, advocacy, and research.	202-223-2226
National Stroke Association 9707 East Easter Lane Englewood, CO 80112 *www.stroke.org*	Their mission is to reduce the incidence and impact of stroke disease and improve quality of patient care and outcomes.	800-787-6537
North American Menopause Society P.O. Box 94527 Cleveland, OH 44101 *www.menopause.org*	Advocacy organization devoted to promoting women's health and quality of life through an understanding of menopause.	440-442-7550
Older Women's League 1750 New York Avenue, NW, Suite 350 Washington, DC 20006 *www.owl-national.org*	Advocacy organization addressing family and caregiver issues.	202-783-6686 800-825-3695

Name & Address	Description	Telephone
Safe Return Alzheimer's Association 225 North Michigan Avenue, Floor 17 Chicago, IL 60601 *www.alz.org*	Joint program of the Alzheimer's Association and the National Center for Missing Persons that provides patients with dementia with a bracelet showing the person's name, the registered caregiver's name, and a toll-free number (800-572-1122) to aid in that person's return, if lost.	888-572-8566
SeniorNet 1171 Homestead Road, Suite 280 Santa Clara, CA 95050 *www.seniornet.com*	National nonprofit organization that works to build a community of computer-using seniors.	408-615-0699
UCLA Center on Aging 10945 Le Conte Avenue, Suite 3119 Los Angeles, CA 90095-6980 *www.aging.ucla.edu*	University center that works to enhance and extend productive and healthy life, through research and education on aging.	310-794-0676
U.S. Dept. of Veterans Affairs 810 Vermont Avenue, NW Washington, DC 20420 *www.va.gov*	Provides information on VA programs, veterans benefits, VA facilities worldwide, and VA medical automation software.	800-827-1000

Bibliography

Agdeppa, E. D., Kepe, V., Petric, A., et al. In vitro detection of (S)-naproxen and ibuprofen binding to plaques in the Alzheimer's brain using the positron emission tomography molecular imaging probe 2-(1-{6-[(2-[^{18}F]fluoro-ethyl)(methyl)amino]-2-naphthyl}ethylidene)malononitrile. *Neuroscience* 117(2003):723–30.

Age-Related Eye Disease Study (AREDS) Research Group. A randomized, placebo-controlled, clinical trial of high-dose supplementation with vitamins C and E and beta carotene for age-related cataract and vision loss: AREDS report no. 9. *Archives of Ophthalmology* 119(2001):1439–52.

Aharon, I., Etcoff, N., Ariely, D., et al. Beautiful faces have variable reward value: fMRI and behavioral evidence. *Neuron* 32(2001):537–51.

Allen, K., Blascovich, J. Effects of music on cardiovascular reactivity among surgeons. *Journal of the American Medical Association* 272(1994):882–4.

Altena, T. S., Michaelson, J. L., Ball, S. D., Thomas, T. R. Single sessions of intermittent and continuous exercise and postprandial lipemia. *Medicine & Science in Sports & Exercise* 36(2004):1364–71.

Andersen, L. D., Remington, P., Trentham-Dietz, A., Reeves, M. Assessing a decade of progress in cancer control. *Oncologist* 7(2002):200–4.

Antell, D. E., Taczanowski, E. M. How environment and lifestyle choices influence the aging process. *Annals of Plastic Surgery* 43(1999):585–8.

Appel, L. J., Champagne, C. M., Harsha, D. W., et al. Effects of comprehensive lifestyle modification on blood pressure control: Main results of the

PREMIER clinical trial. *Journal of the American Medical Association* 289(2003):2083–93.

Arterburn, D. E., Maciejewski, M. L., Tsevat, J. Impact of morbid obesity on medical expenditures in adults. *International Journal of Obesity and Related Metabolic Disorders* 29(2005):334–9.

Ball, K., Berch, D. B., Helmers, K. F., et al. Effects of cognitive training interventions with older adults: A randomized controlled trial. *Journal of the American Medical Association* 288(2002):2271–81.

Barberger-Gateau, P., Letenneur, L., Deschamps, V., et al. Fish, meat, and risk of dementia: Cohort study. *British Medical Journal* 395(2002):932–33.

Bassuk, S. S., Glass, T. A., Berkman, L. F. Social disengagement and incident cognitive decline in community-dwelling elderly persons. *Annals of Internal Medicine* 131(1999):165–73.

Beauchamp, G. K., Keast, R. S., Morel, D., et al. Phytochemistry: Ibuprofen-like activity in extra-virgin olive oil. *Nature* 437(2005):45–6.

Bell, M. L., McDermott, A., Zeger, S. L., Samet, J. M., Dominici, F. Ozone and short-term mortality in 95 U.S. urban communities, 1987–2000. *Journal of the American Medical Association* 292(2004):2372–8.

Bennett, M. P., Zeller, J. M., Rosenberg, L., McCann, J. The effect of mirthful laughter on stress and natural killer cell activity. *Alternative Therapies in Health and Medicine* 9(2003):38–45.

Benson, H. *The Relaxation Response.* New York: Avon, 1975.

Berk, L. S., Tan, S. A., Fry, W. F., et al. Neuroendocrine and stress hormone changes during mirthful laughter. *American Journal of Medical Science* 298(1989):390–6.

Berkowitz, L., Harmon-Jones, E. Toward an understanding of the determinants of anger. *Emotion* 4(2004):107–30.

Berman, B. M., Lao, L., Langenberg, P., et al. Effectiveness of acupuncture as adjunctive therapy in osteoarthritis of the knee: A randomized, controlled trial. *Annals of Internal Medicine* 141(2004):901–10.

Betts, L. R., Taylor, C. P., Sekuler, A. B., Bennett, P. J. Aging reduces center-surround antagonism in visual motion processing. *Neuron* 45(2005):361–6.

Bijlani, R. L., Vempati, R. P., Yadav, R. K., et al. A brief but comprehensive lifestyle education program based on yoga reduces risk factors for cardiovascular disease and diabetes mellitus. *Journal of Alternative and Complementary Medicine* 11(2005):267–74.

Birks J., Grimley Evans, J. Ginkgo biloba for cognitive impairment and dementia (Cochrane Review). The Cochrane Library, Issue 2, 2005. Chichester, U.K.: John Wiley & Sons, Ltd.

Block, J. D. *Sex Over 50*. Paramus, NJ: Reward Books, 1999.

Bone, H. G., Hosking, D., Devogelaer, J. P., et al. Ten years' experience with alendronate for osteoporosis in postmenopausal women. *New England Journal of Medicine* 350(2004):1172–4.

Bookheimer, S. Y., Strojwas, M. H., Cohen, M. S., et al. Brain activation in people at genetic risk for Alzheimer's disease. *New England Journal of Medicine* 343(2000):450–6.

Booth, A., Johnson, D. R., Granger, D. A. Testosterone and men's health. *Journal of Behavioral Medicine* 22(1999):1–19.

Boschmann, M., Steiniger, J., Hille, U., et al. Water-induced thermogenesis. *Journal of Clinical Endocrinology and Metabolism* 88(2003):6015–19.

Bowman, R. E., Beck, K. D., Luine, V. N. Chronic stress effects on memory: Sex differences in performance and monoaminergic activity. *Hormones and Behavior* 43(2003):48–59.

Boyd-Brewer, C., McCaffrey, R. Vibroacoustic sound therapy improves pain management and more. *Holistic Nursing Practice* 18(2004):111–18.

Brand-Miller, J., Volwever, T. M. S., Colaguiri, S., Foster-Powell, K. *The Glucose Revolution*. New York: Marlow & Company, 1999.

Braunstein, G. D., Sundwall, D. A., Katz, M., et al. Safety and efficacy of a testosterone patch for the treatment of hypoactive sexual desire disorder in surgically menopausal women: a randomized, placebo-controlled trial. *Archives of Internal Medicine* 165(2005):1582–9.

Breiter, H. C., Aharon, I., Kahneman, D., Dale, A., Shizgal, P. Functional imaging of neural responses to expectancy and experience of monetary gains and losses. *Neuron* 30(2001):619–39.

Brickman, P., Coates, D., Janoff-Bulman, R. Lottery winners and accident victims: Is happiness relative? *Journal of Personality and Social Psychology* 36(1978):917–27.

Brinkhaus, B., Becker-Witt, C., Jena, S., et al. Acupuncture Randomized Trials (ART) in patients with chronic low back pain and osteoarthritis of the knee—design and protocols. *Forsch Komplementarmed Klass Naturheilkd* 10(2003):185–91.

Brown, K. W., Ryan, R. M. The benefits of being present: Mindfulness and its role in psychological well-being. *Journal of Personality and Social Psychology* 84(2003):822–48.

Calle, E. E., Rodriguez, C., Walker-Thurmond, K., Thun, M. J. Overweight, obesity, and mortality from cancer in a prospectively studied cohort of U.S. adults. *New England Journal of Medicine* 348(2003):1625–38.

Carnethon, M. R., Gidding, S. S., Nehgme, R. et al. Cardiorespiratory fitness in young adulthood and the development of cardiovascular disease risk factors. *Journal of the American Medical Association* 290(2003):3092–100.

Carr, L., Iacoboni, M., Dubeau, M.-C., Mazziotta, J. C., Lenz, G. L. Neural mechanisms of empathy in humans: A relay from neural systems for imitation to limbic areas. *Proceedings of the National Academy of Sciences of the United States of America* 100(2003):5497–5502.

Chafin, S., Roy, M., Gerin, W., Christenfeld, N. Music can facilitate blood pressure recovery from stress. *British Journal of Health and Psychology* 9(2004):393–403.

Chainani-Wu, N. Safety and anti-inflammatory activity of curcumin: A component of tumeric (*Curcuma longa*). *Journal of Alternative and Complementary Medicine* 9(2003):161–8.

Chao, A., Thun, M. J., Connell, C. J., et al. Meat consumption and risk of colorectal cancer. *Journal of the American Medical Association* 293(2005): 172–82.

Chapman, S. B., Weiner, M. F., Rackley, A., Hynan, L. S., Zientz, J. Effects of cognitive-communication stimulation for Alzheimer's disease patients treated with donepezil. *Journal of Speech, Language, and Hearing Research* 47(2004):1149–63.

Charnetski, C. J., Brennan, F. X. Sexual frequency and salivary immunoglobulin A (IgA). *Psychological Reports* 94(2004):839–44.

Chen, J. T., Wesley, R., Shamburek, R. D., Pucino, F., Csako, G. Meta-analysis of natural therapies for hyperlipidemia: Plant sterols and stanols versus policosanol. *Pharmacotherapy* 25(2005):171–83.

Chlebowski, R. T., Wactawski-Wende, J., Ritenbaugh, C., et al. Estrogen plus progestin and colorectal cancer in postmenopausal women. *New England Journal of Medicine* 350(2004):991–1004.

Choi, J. H., Moon, J. S., Song, R. Effects of Sun-style tai chi exercise on physical fitness and fall prevention in fall-prone older adults. *Journal of Advanced Nursing* 51(2005):150–7.

Christensen, H. C., Schüz, J., Kosteljanetz, M., et al. Cellular telephone use and risk of acoustic neuroma. *American Journal of Epidemiology* 159(2004):277–83.

Clark, A., Seidler, A., Miller, M. Inverse association between sense of humor and coronary heart disease. *International Journal of Cardiology* 80(2001):87–8.

Clark, N. *Nancy Clark's Sports Nutrition Guidebook*, Third Edition. Champaign, IL: Human Kinetics Publishing, 2003.

Colcombe, S. J., Erickson, K. I., Raz, N., et al. Aerobic fitness reduces brain tissue loss in aging humans. *Journal of Gerontology: Biological Sciences and Medical Sciences* 58A(2003):176–80.

Contento, I. R., Basch, C., Zybert, P. Body image, weight, and food choices of Latina women and their young children. *Journal of Nutrition Education and Behavior* 35(2003):236–48.

Dahlberg, L. L., Ikeda, R. M., and Kresnow, M. Guns in the home and risk of a violent death in the home: Findings from a national study. *American Journal of Epidemiology* 160(2004):929–36.

Dallongeville, J., Marecaux, N., Ducimetiere, P., et al. Influence of alcohol consumption and various beverages on waist girth and waist-to-hip ratio in a sample of French men and women. *International Journal of Obesity and Related Metabolic Disorders* 22(1998):1178–83.

Davey Smith, G., Frankel, S., Yarnell, J. Sex and death: are they related? Findings from the Caerphilly Cohort Study. *British Medical Journal* 315(1997):1641–4.

Davidson, R. J., Kabat-Zinn, J., Schumacher, J., et al. Alterations in brain and immune function produced by mindfulness meditation. *Psychosomatic Medicine* 65(2003):564–70.

de Castro, J. M. The time of day of food intake influences overall intake in humans. *The Journal of Nutrition* 134(2004):104–11.

de Lorgeril, M., Salen, P., Martin, J.-L., et al. Mediterranean diet, traditional risk factors, and the rate of cardiovascular complications after myocardial infarction: Final report of the Lyon Diet Heart Study. *Circulation* 99 (1999):779–85.

De Smet, P. Herbal remedies. *New England Journal of Medicine* 347(2002):2046–56.

Del Ser, T., Hachinski, V., Merskey, H., Munoz, D. G. An autopsy-verified study of the effect of education on degenerative dementia. *Brain* 122(1999):2309–19.

Dickey, R. A., Janick, J. J. Lifestyle modifications in the prevention and treatment of hypertension. *Endocrine Practice* 7(2001):392–9.

Doerksen, S., Shimamura, A. P. Source memory enhancement for emotional words. *Emotion* 1(2001):5–11.

Draganski, B., Gaser, C., Busch, V., et al. Neuroplasticity: Changes in grey matter induced by training. *Nature* 427(2004):311–12.

Eckman, P. *Emotions Revealed: Recognizing Faces and Feelings to Improve Communication and Emotional Life*. New York: Times Books, 2003.

Ehlenfeldt, M. K., Prior, R. L. Oxygen Radical Absorbance Capacity (ORAC) and phenolic and anthocyanin concentrations in fruit and leaf tissues of highbush blueberry. *Journal of Agriculture and Food Chemistry* 49(2001): 2222–7.

Eng, P. M., Fitzmaurice, G., Kubzansky, L. D., Rimm, E. B., Kawachi, I. Anger expression and risk of stroke and coronary heart disease among male health professionals. *Psychosomatic Medicine* 65(2003):100–10.

Epel, E. S., Blackburn, E. H., Lin, J., et al. Accelerated telomere shortening in response to life stress. *Proceedings of the National Academy of Sciences of the United States of America.* 101(2004):17312–15.

Eriksson, J., Lindstrom, J., Tuomilehto, J. Potential for the prevention of type 2 diabetes. *British Medical Bulletin* 60(2001):183–99.

Evans, J. R. Ginkgo biloba extract for age-related macular degeneration (Cochrane Review). The Cochrane Library, Issue 4, 2005. Chichester, UK: John Wiley & Sons, Ltd.

Fairfield, K. M., Fletcher, R. H. Vitamins for chronic disease prevention in adults: Scientific review. *Journal of the American Medical Association* 287(2002):3116–26.

Fajardo, M., Di Cesare, P. E. Disease-modifying therapies for osteoarthritis: Current status. *Drugs & Aging* 22(2005):141–61.

Fan, J., Liu, F., Wu, J., Dai, W. Visual perception of female physical attractiveness. *Proceedings of the Royal Society of London* 271(2004):347–52.

Feldman, H. A., Johannes, C. B., McKinlay, J. B., Longcope, C. Low dehydroepiandrosterone sulfate and heart disease in middle-aged men: Cross-sectional results from the Massachusetts Male Aging Study. *Annals of Epidemiology* 8(1998):217–28.

Feldman, S. R., Liguori, A., Kucenic, M., et al. Ultraviolet exposure is a reinforcing stimulus in frequent indoor tanners. *Journal of the American Academy of Dermatology* 51(2004):45–51.

Ferro, A. R., Kopperud, R. J., Hildemann, L. M. Source strengths for indoor human activities that resuspend particulate matter. *Environmental Science & Technology* 38(2004):1759–64.

Fonarow, G. C., Wright, R. S., Spencer, F. A., et al. Effect of statin use within the first 24 hours of admission for acute myocardial infarction on early morbidity and mortality. *American Journal of Cardiology* 96(2005):611–16.

Frank, L. D., Andresen, M. A., Schmid, T. L. Obesity relationships with community design, physical activity, and time spent in cars. *American Journal of Preventive Medicine* 27(2004):87–96.

Fraser, G. E., Shavlik, D. J. Ten years of life: Is it a matter of choice? *Archives of Internal Medicine* 161(2001):1645–52.

Gadek-Michalska, A., Bugajski, J. Repeated handling, restraint, or chronic crowding impair the hypothalamic-pituitary-adrenocortical response to acute restraint stress. *Journal of Physiological Pharmacology* 54(2003): 449–59.

Gage, F. H. Neurogenesis in the adult brain. *Journal of Neuroscience* 22(2002):612–13.

Gauderman, W. J., Avol, E., Gilliland, F., et al. The effect of air pollution on lung development from 10 to 18 years of age. *New England Journal of Medicine* 351(2004):1057–67.

Geday, J., Gjedde, A., Boldsen, A.-S., Kupers, R. Emotional valence modulates activity in the posterior fusiform gyrus and inferior medial prefrontal cortex in social perception. *NeuroImage* 18(2003):675–84.

Gilewski, M. J., Zelinski, E. M., Schaie, K. W. The Memory Functioning Questionnaire for assessment of memory complaints in adulthood and old age. *Psychology and Aging* 5(1990):482–90.

Glass, T. A., de Leon, C. M., Marottoli, R. A., Berkman, L. F. Population based study of social and productive activities as predictors of survival among elderly Americans. *British Medical Journal* 319(1999):478–83.

Green, C. S., Bavelier, D. Action video game modifies visual selective attention. *Nature* 423(2003):534–7.

Greenblatt, D. Treatment of postmenopausal osteoporosis. *Pharmacotherapy* 25(2005):574–84.

Gurung, R. A., Taylor, S. E., Seeman, T. E. Accounting for changes in social support among married older adults: Insights from the MacArthur Studies of Successful Aging. *Psychology and Aging* 18(2003):487–96.

Hathcock, J. N. Vitamins and minerals: Efficacy and safety. *American Journal of Clinical Nutrition* 66(1997):427–37.

Hayashi, K., Hayashi, T., Iwanaga, S., et al. Laughter lowered the increase in postprandial blood glucose. *Diabetes Care* 26(2003):1651–2.

He, F. J., MacGregor, G. A. Effect of modest salt reduction on blood pressure: A meta-analysis of randomized trials. Implications for public health. *Journal of Human Hypertension* 16(2002):761–70.

Heart Protection Study Collaborative Group. MRC/BHF Heart Protection Study of cholesterol lowering with simvastatin in 20,536 high-risk individuals: A randomized placebo-controlled trial. *Lancet* 360(2002):7–22.

Heber, D., Bowerman, S. *What Color Is Your Diet?* New York: Regan Books, 2001.

Heisler, M., Langa, K. M., Eby, E. L., et al. The health effects of restricting prescription medication use because of cost. *Medical Care* 42(2004):626–34.

Henwood, T. R., Taaffe, D. R. Improved physical performance in older adults undertaking a short-term programme of high-velocity resistance training. *Gerontology* 51(2005):108–15.

Hightower, J. M., Moore, D. Mercury levels in high-end consumers of fish. *Environmental Health Perspective* 111(2003):604–8.

Horwich, T. B., MacLellan, W. R., Fonarow, G. C. Statin therapy is associated with improved survival in ischemic and non-ischemic heart failure. *Journal of the American College of Cardiology* 43(2004):642–8.

Hui, K. K., Liu, J., Makris, N., et al. Acupuncture modulates the limbic system and subcortical gray structures of the human brain: Evidence from fMRI studies in normal subjects. *Human Brain Mapping* 9(2000):13–25.

Hummer, R. A., Rogers, R. G., Nam, C. B., Ellison, C. G. Religious involvement and U.S. adult mortality. *Demography* 36(1999):273–85.

Irwin, M. R., Pike, J. L., Cole, J. C., Oxman, M. N. Effects of a behavioral intervention, tai chi chih, on varicella-zoster virus specific immunity and health functioning in older adults. *Psychosomatic Medicine* 65(2003): 824–30.

Järvinen, R., Knekt, P., Hakulinen, T., Aromaa, A. Prospective study on milk products, calcium, and cancers of the colon and rectum. *Journal of the National Cancer Institute* 55(2001):1000–7.

Johnson, S. M. The revolution in couple therapy: A practitioner-scientist perspective. *Journal of Marital and Family Therapy* 29(2003):365–84.

Joseph, J. A., Nadeau, D., Underwood, A. *The Color Code: A Revolutionary Eating Plan for Optimum Health.* New York: Hyperion, 2002.

Kabat-Zinn, J., Lipworth, L., Burney, R., Sellers, W. Four year follow-up of a meditation-based program for the self-regulation of chronic pain: Treatment outcomes and compliance. *Clinical Journal of Pain* 2(1986):159–73.

Kabat-Zinn, J., Massion, A. O., Kristeller, J., et al. Effectiveness of a meditation-based stress reduction program in the treatment of anxiety disorders. *American Journal of Psychiatry* 149(1992):936–43.

Kabat-Zinn, J., Wheeler, E., Light, T., et al. Influence of a mindfulness-based stress reduction intervention on rates of skin clearing in patients with moderate to severe psoriasis undergoing phototherapy (UVB) and photochemotherapy (PUVA). *Psychosomatic Medicine* 60(1998):625–32.

Kahn, R. L., Rowe, J. W. *Successful Aging.* New York: Pantheon, 1998.

Karlin, W. A., Brondolo, E., Schwartz, J. Workplace social support and ambulatory cardiovascular activity in New York City traffic agents. *Psychosomatic Medicine* 65(2003):167–76.

Karvonen, M. J. Sports and longevity. *Advances in Cardiology* 18(1976):243–8.

Kiecolt-Glaser, J. K., Preacher, K. J., MacCallum, R. C., et al. Chronic stress and age-related increases in the proinflammatory cytokine IL-6. *Proceedings of the National Academy of Sciences of the United States of America* 100(2003):9090–5.

Knoops, K.T.B., de Groot, L.C., Kromhout, D., et al. Mediterranean diet, lifestyle factors, and 10-year mortality in elderly European men and women. *Journal of the American Medical Association* 292(2004):1433–9.

Koenig, H.G., George, L.K., Titus, P. Religion, spirituality, and health in medically ill hospitalized older patients. *Journal of the American Geriatrics Society* 52(2004):554–62.

Kousa, A., Moltchanova, E., Viik-Kajander, M., et al. Geochemistry of ground water and the incidence of acute myocardial infarction in Finland. *Journal of Epidemiology and Community Health* 58(2004):136–9.

Kubey, R., Csikszentmihalyi, M. Television addiction is no mere metaphor. *Scientific American* 286(2002):74–80.

Kwallek, N., Lewis, C.M. Effects of environmental colour on males and females: A red or white or green office. *Applied Ergonomics* 21(1990):275–8.

Law, M., Wald, N., Morris, J. Lowering blood pressure to prevent myocardial infarction and stroke: A new preventive strategy. *Health Technology Assessment* 7(2003):1–94.

Lazar, S.W., Bush, G., Gollub, R.L., et al. Functional brain mapping of the relaxation response and meditation. *Neuroreport* 11(2000):1581–5.

Lee, I.M., Cook, N.R. Gaziano, J.M., et al. Vitamin E in the primary prevention of cardiovascular disease and cancer: The Women's Health Study: A randomized controlled trial. *Journal of the American Medical Association* 294(2005):56–65.

Lee, I.M., Hsieh, C.C., Paffenbarger, R.S. Exercise intensity and longevity in men. *Journal of the American Medical Association* 273(1995):1179–84.

Lee, I.M., Sesso, H.D., Oguma, Y., Paffenbarger, R.S. Jr. The "weekend warrior" and risk of mortality. *American Journal of Epidemiology* 160(2004):636–41.

Leetun, D.T., Ireland, M.L., Willson, J.D., Ballantyne, B.T., Davis, I.M. Core stability measures as risk factors for lower extremity injury in athletes. *Medicine & Science in Sports & Exercise* 36(2004):926–34.

Lim, G.P., Chu, T., Yang, F., Beech, W., Frautschy, S.A., Cole, G.M. The curry spice curcumin reduces oxidative damage and amyloid pathology in an Alzheimer transgenic mouse. *Journal of Neuroscience* 21(2001):8370–7.

Liu, S., Manson, J.E., Stampfer, M.J., et al. Whole-grain consumption and risk of ischemic stroke in women: A prospective study. *Journal of the American Medical Association* 284(2000):1534–40.

Liu-Ambrose, T., Khan, K. M., Eng, J. J., Janssen, P. A., Lord, S. R., McKay, H. A. Resistance and agility training reduce fall risk in women aged 75 to 85 with low bone mass: A 6-month randomized, controlled trial. *Journal of the American Geriatrics Society* 52(2004):657–65.

Loewenstein, D. A., Acevedo, A., Czaja, S. J., Duara, R. Cognitive rehabilitation of mildly impaired Alzheimer disease patients on cholinesterase inhibitors. *American Journal of Geriatric Psychiatry* 12(2004):395–402.

Ma, Y., Bertone, E. R., Stanek, E. J., III, et al. Association between eating patterns and obesity in a free-living U.S. adult population. *American Journal of Epidemiology* 158(2003):85–92.

MacDonald, G. *Massage for the Hospital Patient and Medically Frail Client.* New York: Lippincott Williams & Wilkins, 2004.

Maguire, E. A., Valentine, E. R., Wilding, J. M., Kapur, N. Routes to remembering: The brains behind superior memory. *Nature Neuroscience* 6(2003):90–5.

Malliaropoulos, N., Papalexandris, S., Papalada, A., Papacostas, E. The role of stretching in rehabilitation of hamstring injuries: 80 athletes follow-up. *Medicine & Science in Sports & Exercise* 36(2004):756–9.

McClure, S. M., Laibson, D. I., Loewenstein, G., Cohen, J. D. Separate neural systems value immediate and delayed monetary rewards. *Science* 306(2004):503–7.

McEwen, B. *The End of Stress As We Know It.* Washington, DC: The Dana Press, 2004.

Means, K. M., Rodell, D. E., O'Sullivan, P. S. Balance, mobility, and falls among community-dwelling elderly persons: Effects of a rehabilitation exercise program. *American Journal of Physical Medicine & Rehabilitation* 84(2005):238–50.

Menec, V. H. The relation between everyday activities and successful aging: A 6-year longitudinal study. *Journal of Gerontology Series B: Psychological Sciences and Social Sciences* 58(2003):S74–S82.

Miller, E. R., Pastor-Barriuso, R., Dalal, D., et al. Meta-analysis: High-dosage vitamin E supplementation may increase all-cause mortality. *Annals of Internal Medicine* 142(2005):37–46.

Moore, A. A., Gould, R., Reuben, D. B., et al. Longitudinal patterns and predictors of alcohol consumption in the United States. *American Journal of Public Health* 95(2005):458–65.

Morris, M. C., Evans, D. A., Bienias, J. L., et al. Dietary niacin and the risk of incident Alzheimer's disease and of cognitive decline. *Journal of Neurology, Neurosurgery and Psychiatry* 75(2004):1093–99.

Mukamal, K. J., Kuller, L. H., Fitzpatrick, A. L., et al. Prospective study of alcohol consumption and risk of dementia in older adults. *Journal of the American Medical Association* 289(2003):1405–13.

Murtaugh, M. A., Jacobs, D. R. Jr., Jacob, B., Steffen, L. M., Marquart, L. Epidemiological support for the protection of whole grains against diabetes. *The Proceedings of the Nutrition Society* 62(2003):143–9.

Newberg, A., Alavi, A., Baime, M., Pourdehnad, M., Santanna, J., d'Aquili, E. The measurement of regional cerebral blood flow during the complex cognitive task of meditation: A preliminary SPECT study. *Psychiatry Research* 106(2001):113–22.

Nissen, S. E., Tuzcu, E. M., Libby, P., et al. Effect of antihypertensive agents on cardiovascular events in patients with coronary disease and normal blood pressure: The CAMELOT study: A randomized controlled trial. *Journal of the American Medical Association* 292(2004):2217–25.

North American Menopause Society. Recommendations for estrogen and progestogen use in peri- and postmenopausal women: October 2004 position statement of The North American Menopause Society. *Menopause* 11(2004):589–600.

Olshansky, J., Passaro, D. J., Hershow, R. C., et al. A potential decline in life expectancy in the United States in the 21st century. *New England Journal of Medicine* 352(2005):1138–45.

Paffenbarger, R. S. Jr., Hyde, R. T., Wing, A. L., Hsieh, C. C. Physical activity, all-cause mortality, and longevity of college alumni. *New England Journal of Medicine* 314(1986):605–13.

Palmore, E. Predictors of the longevity difference: A 25-year follow-up. *Gerontologist* 22(1982):513–18.

Pargament, K. I., Koenig, H. G., Tarakeshwar, N., Hahn, J. Religious struggle as a predictor of mortality among medically ill elderly patients: a 2-year longitudinal study. *Archives of Internal Medicine* 161(2001):1881–5.

Pate, R. R., Pratt, M., Blair, S. N., et al. Physical activity and public health. A recommendation from the Centers for Disease Control and Prevention and the American College of Sports Medicine. *Journal of the American Medical Association* 273(1995):402–7.

Persson, G. Five-year mortality in a 70-year-old urban population in relation to psychiatric diagnosis, personality, sexuality and early parental death. *Journal of Psychosomatic Research* 24(1980):244–53.

Peters, A., von Klot, S., Heier, M., et al. Exposure to traffic and the onset of myocardial infarction. *New England Journal of Medicine* 351(2004):1721–30.

Petersen, R. C., Thomas, R. G., Grundman, M., et al. Vitamin E and donepezil for the treatment of mild cognitive impairment. *New England Journal of Medicine* 352(2005):2379–88.

Pew Internet & American Life Project. *The Internet and Daily Life.* 2004. http://www.pewinternet.org/

Poynter, J. N., Gruber, S. B., Higgins, P. D., et al. Statins and the risk of colorectal cancer. *New England Journal of Medicine* 352(2005):2184–92.

Prigerson, H. G., Maciejewski, P. K., Rosenheck, R. A. The effects of marital dissolution and marital quality on health and health service use among women. *Medical Care* 37(1999):858–73.

Rami, T., Shih, H. T. Update of implantable cardioverter/defibrillator and cardiac resynchronization therapy in heart failure. *Current Opinions in Cardiology* 19(2004):264–9.

Raskind, M. A., Peskind, E. R., Wessel, T., and the Galantamine USA-1 Study Group. Galantamine in AD. A 6-month randomized, placebo-controlled trial with a 6-month extension. *Neurology* 54(2000):2269–2276.

Rea, T. D., Breitner, J. C., Psaty, B. M., et al. Statin use and the risk of incident dementia: The Cardiovascular Health Study. *Archives of Neurology* 62(2005):1047–51.

Reisberg, B., Doody, R., Stoffler, A., et al. Memantine in moderate-to-severe Alzheimer's disease. *New England Journal of Medicine* 348(2003): 1333–41.

Rennie, M. J. Claims for the anabolic effects of growth hormone: A case of the Emperor's new clothes? *British Journal of Sports Medicine* 37(2003): 100–5.

Rimm, E. B., Ascherio, A., Giovannucci, E., et al. Vegetable, fruit, and cereal fiber intake and risk of coronary heart disease among men. *Journal of the American Medical Association* 275(1996):447–51.

Rimm, E. B., Stampfer, M. J. Diet, lifestyle, and longevity—The next steps? *Journal of the American Medical Association* 292(2004):1490–2.

Rozmus-Wrzesinska, M., Pawlowski, B. Men's ratings of female attractiveness are influenced more by changes in female waist size compared with changes in hip size. *Biological Psychology* 68(2005):299–308.

Ruitenberg, A., van Swieten, J. C., Witteman, J. C., et al. Alcohol consumption and risk of dementia: The Rotterdam Study. *Lancet* 359(2002):281–6.

Sano, M., Ernesto, C., Thomas, R. G., et al. A controlled trial of selegiline, alpha-tocopherol, or both as treatment for Alzheimer's disease. *New England Journal of Medicine* 336(1997):1216–22.

Schneider, R. H., Alexander, C. N., Staggers, F., et al. A randomized controlled trial of stress reduction in African Americans treated for hypertension for over one year. *American Journal of Hypertension* 18(2005):88–98.

Schneider, R. H., Alexander, C. N., Staggers, F., et al. Long-term effects of stress reduction on mortality in persons > or = 55 years of age with systemic hypertension. *American Journal of Cardiology* 95(2005):1060–4.

Sesso, H. D., Chen, R. S., L'Italien, G. J., et al. Blood pressure lowering and life expectancy based on a Markov model of cardiovascular events. *Hypertension* 42(2003):885–90.

Shenk, D. *Data Smog: Surviving the Information Glut.* New York: HarperCollins, 1997.

Sherman, S. E., D'Agostino, R. B., Cobb, J. L., Kannel, W. B. Physical activity and mortality in women in the Framingham Heart Study. *American Heart Journal* 128(1994):879–84.

Shoghi-Jadid, K., Small, G. W., Agdeppa, E. D., et al. Localization of neurofibrillary tangles and beta-amyloid plaques in the brains of living patients with Alzheimer disease. *American Journal of Geriatric Psychiatry* 10(2002): 24–35.

Shumaker, S. A., Legault, C., Rapp, S. R., et al. Estrogen plus progestin and the incidence of dementia and mild cognitive impairment in postmenopausal women. The Women's Health Initiative Memory Study: A randomized controlled trial. *Journal of the American Medical Association* 289(2003):2651–62.

Simon, S. R., Chan, K. A., Soumerai, S. B., et al. Potentially inappropriate medication use by elderly persons in U.S. Health Maintenance Organizations, 2000–2001. *Journal of the American Geriatric Society* 53 (2005): 227–32.

Singer, T., Seymour, B., O'Doherty, J., Kaube, H., Dolan, R. J., Frith, C. D. Empathy for pain involves the affective but not sensory components of pain. *Science* 303(2004):1157–62.

Small, G., Vorgan G. *The Memory Prescription: Dr. Gary Small's 14-Day Plan to Keep Your Brain and Body Young.* New York: Hyperion, 2004.

Small, G. *The Memory Bible: An Innovative Strategy for Keeping Your Brain Young.* New York: Hyperion, 2002.

Small, G. W., Silverman, D. H., Siddarth, P., et al. Brain function and physical effects of a 14-day healthy lifestyle program. *9th International Conference on Alzheimer's Disease and Related Disorders,* 2004.

Small, G. W. What we need to know about age related memory loss. *British Medical Journal* 324(2002):1502–5.

Smith, G. D., Frankel, S., Yarnell, J. Sex and death, are they related? Findings from the Caerphilly cohort study. *British Medical Journal* 315(1997): 164–5.

Soeken, K. L., Lee, W. L., Bausell, R. B., Agelli, M., Berman, B. M. Safety and efficacy of S-adenosylmethionine (SAMe) for osteoarthritis. *Journal of Family Practice* 51(2002):425–30.

Spiro, H. What is empathy and can it be taught? *Annals of Internal Medicine* 116(1992):843–6.

Springer, M. V., McIntosh, A. R., Winocur, G., Grady, C. L. The relation between brain activity during memory tasks and years of education in young and older adults. *Neuropsychology* 19(2005):181–92.

Stanton, R., Reaburn, P. R., Humphries, B. The effect of short-term Swiss ball training on core stability and running economy. *Journal of Strength and Conditioning Research* 18(2004):522–8.

Stevens, C., Tiggemann, M. Women's body figure preferences across the life span. *Journal of Genetic Psychology* 159(1998):94–102.

Takahashi, M., Nakata, A., Haratani, T., Ogawa, Y., Arito, H. Post-lunch nap as a worksite intervention to promote alertness on the job. *Ergonomics* 47 (2004):1003–13.

Takano, T., Nakamura, K., Watanabe, M. Urban residential environments and senior citizens' longevity in megacity areas: The importance of walkable green spaces. *Journal of Epidemiology and Community Health* 56(2002):913–18.

Thomsen, D. K., Mehlsen, M. Y., Hokland, M., et al. Negative thoughts and health: Associations among rumination, immunity, and health care utilization in a young and elderly sample. *Psychosomatic Medicine* 66(2004): 363–71.

Travis, F., Arenander, A., DuBois, D. Psychological and physiological characteristics of a proposed object-referral/self-referral continuum of self-awareness. *Consciousness Cognition* 13(2004):401–20.

Turner, R. B., Bauer, R., Woelkart, K., Hulsey, T. C., Gangemi, J. D. An evaluation of *Echinacea angustifolia* in experimental rhinovirus infections. *New England Journal of Medicine* 353(2005):341–8.

USC Annenberg School Center for the Digital Future. *The Digital Future Report.* 2004. http://www.digitalcenter.org/

van der Valk, R., Webers, C. A., Schouten, J. S., et al. Intraocular pressure-lowering effects of all commonly used glaucoma drugs: A meta-analysis of randomized clinical trials. *Ophthalmology* 112(2005):1177–85.

Van Gaal, L. F., Rissanen, A. M., Scheen, A. J., et al. Effects of the cannabinoid-1 receptor blocker rimonabant on weight reduction and cardiovascular risk factors in overweight patients: 1-year experience from the RIO-Europe study. *Lancet* 365(2005):1389–97.

Verghese, J., Lipton, R. B., Katz, M. J., et al. Leisure activities and the risk of dementia in the elderly. *New England Journal of Medicine* 348(2003): 2508–16.

Verhagen, E., van der Beek, A., Twisk, J., Bouter, L., Bahr, R., van Mechelen, W. The effect of a proprioceptive balance board training program for the prevention of ankle sprains: A prospective controlled trial. *American Journal of Sports Medicine* 32(2004):1385–93.

Vermeire, K., Brokx, J. P., Wuyts, F. L., et al. Quality-of-life benefit from cochlear implantation in the elderly. *Otology & Neurotology* 26(2005): 188–95.

Vijan, S., Hayward, R. A.; American College of Physicians. Pharmacologic lipid-lowering therapy in type 2 diabetes mellitus: Background paper for the American College of Physicians. *Annals of Internal Medicine* 140(2004): 650–8.

Villareal, D. T., Holloszy, J. O. Effect of DHEA on abdominal fat and insulin action in elderly women and men: A randomized controlled trial. *Journal of the American Medical Association* 292(2004):2243–8.

Wager, N., Fieldman, G., Hussey, T. The effect on ambulatory blood pressure of working under favourably and unfavourably perceived supervisors. *Journal of Occupational and Environmental Medicine* 60(2003):468–74.

Wang Y., Wang, Q. J. The prevalence of prehypertension and hypertension among U.S. adults according to the new joint national committee guidelines: New challenges of the old problem. *Archives of Internal Medicine* 164(2004):2126–34.

Wannamethee, S. G., Camargo, C. A. Jr., Manson, J. E., Willett, W. C., Rimm, E. B. Alcohol drinking patterns and risk of type 2 diabetes mellitus among younger women. *Archives of Internal Medicine* 163(2003): 1329–36.

Wansink B., Lee, K. Cooking habits provide a key to 5 a day success. *Journal of the American Dietetic Association* 104(2004):1648–50.

Wansink, B., Linder, L. R. Interactions between forms of fat consumption and restaurant bread consumption. *International Journal of Obesity* 27(2003): 866–8.

Weuve, J., Kang, J. H., Manson, J. E., et al. Physical activity, including walking, and cognitive function in older women. *Journal of the American Medical Association* 292(2004):1454–61.

Williams, F. M., Cherkas, L. F., Spector, T. D., MacGregor, A. J. The effect of moderate alcohol consumption on bone mineral density: A study of female twins. *Annals of the Rheumatic Diseases* 64(2005):309–10.

Wilson, R. S., Evans, D. A., Bienias, J. L., et al. Proneness to psychological distress is associated with risk of Alzheimer's disease. *Neurology* 61(2003): 1479–85.

Zelinski, E. M., Gilewski, M. J., Anthony-Bergstone, C. R. Memory Functioning Questionnaire: Concurrent validity with memory performance and self-reported memory failures. *Psychology and Aging* 5(1990):388–99.

Index

abdominal exercises, 159–60
  crunch, 178–79
  side toning, 179
acetaminophen, 220
acetylcholine, 221
Achilles tendon stretch, 165–66
Actonel, 217
acupuncture, 106–7
adult children and their parents, 71,
  85–87, 138–39
adversity, 46–47
Advil, 192, 220
aerobics classes, 153
Aeschylus, 15
aesthetic living, 117–19
Aharon, Itzhak, 147
air, 132–34
Albright, Herm, 43
alcoholic beverages, 186–87
  bone health and, 217
alendronate, 217
Aleve, 193, 220
allergies, 113, 133, 134
  bedding and, 120
alternating overhead stretch, 162
Alzheimer's disease, 5, 11, 16, 17, 24, 29
  coenzyme Q_{10} and, 230

dancing and, 153
diet and, 190, 192
free radicals and, 190
ginkgo biloba and, 232
gum disease and, 246
medications and, 192–93
omega-3 fats and, 192, 231
physical activity and, 145
prevention and treatment of, 29–30,
  219, 221–23, 231
stress and, 62, 91
vitamins and, 229, 230
amino acids, 185, 190–92, 199, 236
amitriptyline, 224
anger, 101–2
  letting go of, 57–58, 79, 103
angioplasty, 210
Antell, Darrick, 135
antihistamines, 213
antioxidants, 184, 185, 190, 191, 200,
  225, 229–30, 231
apartments, toxins in, 133
appetite, 91, 209
  sleep and, 119
apple crumble à la mode, 263
Aricept, 29, 30, 221, 222
arm stretch, 175–76

Index

art, 20, 47, 118, 119
arthritis
  acupuncture and, 107
  diet and, 193
  driving and, 137
  exercise and, 157
  free radicals and, 190
  mindful awareness and, 8
  treatment of, 219–20, 232, 233
aspirin, 213, 232–33
assisted living, 139
asthma, 132, 133, 134
attentive listening, 74–76
Avandia, 218

back leg lift, 180
back pain, 78, 113, 120, 159–60
balance, 154–55, 159
balance and flexibility work, 7, 149,
  154–57, 158, 160, 217
  dancing and, 153
  strengthening, 161–82
  tai chi, 113, 155–56
balance boards, 157
Baltimore Longitudinal Study of Aging,
  11
bean, white, salad, 270
beans, green, with lemon, 266–67
beauty, see youthfulness and
  attractiveness
bedding, 120
bedrooms, 105, 118, 119–21
Benadryl, 213
Benson, Herbert, 95
beta carotene, 230–31
Bextra, 220
biceps curl, 170–71
bicycling, 133, 137, 150, 152–53
  stationary, 153, 154
bimatoprost, 226
blood pressure
  antidepressants and, 224
  normal, guidelines for, 216
  see also high blood pressure
blood sugar, 212, 218
  exercise and, 157
  glycemic index and, 195, 196–97, 199

bones, 145, 157, 192, 216–17
Botox injections, 241
brain, 185, 186
  anger and, 101–2
  building mass of, 21–23
  connections in, 17, 21
  cross-training, 30
  curcumin and, 231
  empathy hardwired in, 71–72
  financial decisions and, 107–8
  meditation and, 94
  multitasking and, 97
  prefrontal cortex of, 97, 107
  right and left sides of, 20
  see also mental sharpness
breast lifts, 239
Brondolo, Elizabeth, 62
Buber, Martin, 8
buttermilk dressing, lowfat, 264
bypass surgery, 210

caffeine, 105, 111
cake, 184, 187
calcitonin, 217
calcium, 192, 217, 221
calf strengthener, 170
calories, 77, 150, 154, 157, 187–88, 193
cancer, 7, 48, 210, 211
  curcumin and, 231
  diet and, 184, 185, 192, 193, 196
  free radicals and, 190
  hormone therapies and, 234, 235
  meditation and, 95
  physical activity and, 145
  smoking and, 135
  stress and, 91
  sun exposure and, 136
  treatments for, 211, 219
  vitamins and, 229, 230
  wine and, 187
carbohydrates, 184, 185, 186, 187, 198,
  199
  glycemic index and, 195, 196–97, 199
  whole grains, 185, 194–98, 199, 200
cardiovascular conditioning, 7, 149,
  150–54, 158, 161
cardiovascular disease, see heart disease

Index

Index

noise, 118
  in bedroom, 118, 120–21
  hearing problems from, 131–32, 226
  in workplace, 131–32
NSAIDs (nonsteroidal anti-inflammatory
  drugs), 220
nursing homes, 139
nutrition, see diet; Longevity Diet
nuts, 185, 194, 200

olive oil, 184, 192, 193, 200
omega-3 fats, 185, 192, 193, 200
  supplements of, 231–32
onion
  caramelized, dip, 264
  fennel, and orange salad, 266
optimism, see positive outlook
orange, fennel, and red onion salad, 266
organization, 110, 128
  clutter and, 7, 114, 121–23, 124, 128,
    138, 140, 141, 252
  multitasking and, 96–98
organizations, 279–87
osteoarthritis, 219–20
  see also arthritis
osteoporosis, 157, 216–17
overhead press, 174
overhead stretch exercise, 162

pain, 6, 223
  acupuncture and, 106–7
  back, 78, 113, 120, 159–60
  exercise and, 159–61
  mindful awareness and, 8
  pets and, 85
  positive outlook and, 44
  relationships and, 62
  self-hypnosis and, 113
  sound and, 118
parents and adult children, 71, 85–87,
    138–39
Pargament, Kenneth, 48
paroxetine, 224
pasta
  cheesy pesto with, 265
  mixed seafood and linguini, 267
Pavlov, Ivan, 129

Paxil, 224
pea soup, lowfat split, 269
pelvic tilt, 179–80
perseverance, in mental sharpness,
  18–19
pesto with pasta, cheesy, 265
pets, 85
photofacial, 244
physical activity, 144–45
  housework and gardening, 154
  sleep and, 106
  stress and, 113–14
  see also fitness and exercise
Pilates, 148, 149, 156, 160
pillows, 120
policosanol, 233
pollution, 116, 132–33
positive outlook, 5–6, 11, 19, 43–59, 79,
  236, 252
  checklist for working on, 254–55
  dealing with negative thoughts and
    feelings, 52–57
  forgiveness in, 57–58
  happiness in, 46–47
  mindful awareness and, 9, 94
  self-confidence in, see self-confidence
    and self-esteem
  setting goals for working on, 261–62
  spirituality and religion in, 9, 44,
    47–49
  stress and, 91
poultry, 184, 191, 193, 194
prayer, 48, 49
presence and focus, in mental sharpness,
  18–19, 25, 97, 113
procrastination, 110
progestin, 234
Propecia, 246
proprioception, 154–55
Proscar, 246
proteins, 185, 190–92, 194, 199, 200
  complete and incomplete, 191–92
Prozac, 224
puzzles and mental aerobics, 5, 9,
  15–16, 17, 20, 21, 22, 23, 30–41,
  96, 271–78
  lateral thinking and, 30

Index

Shakespeare, William, 208
shoulder stretch, 175
side stretch, 162–63
Singer, Tania, 72
single people, happiness and, 84
skin
    creams for, 245
    smoking and, 135
    sun exposure and, 136, 236
    see also cosmetic medicine
sleep, 104–6, 119
    bedding and, 120
    getting too much, 119
    light and, 120
    mattress and, 119–20
    naps, 105, 111–12
    noise and, 118, 120–21
    reading and, 105, 121
    sex and, 78
    snacking and, 186
    television and, 105, 121
    temperature and, 121
smoking, 134–35
snacks, 186
Snap, in memory technique, 24, 25–28
socializing, 61–62, 113–14
    marriage and, 83–84
    see also relationships
sorbet, strawberry, 270
soups
    five-minute fat-free chilled strawberry, 265–66
    split pea, lowfat, 269
soybeans, 191–92, 194
spinning classes, 152–53
spirituality and religion, 9, 44, 47–49
    sexual activity and, 78
Spitz, Rene, 61
stability balls, 156–57
statin drugs, 8, 210–11, 219
stem cells, 209
step and stair-climbing machines, 150, 154
strawberry
    sorbet, 270
    soup, five-minute fat-free chilled, 265–66

strength training, 7, 149, 157–59, 161–82
stress, 5, 6, 9, 11, 89–115, 141, 252
    acupuncture and, 106–7
    anger and, 101–2
    checklist for dealing with, 256
    clutter and, 7, 121
    driving and, 137
    exercise and, 91, 150
    financial worries and, 107–9
    forgiveness and, 57
    laughter and, 103
    meditation and, 48, 49
    mindful awareness and, 8, 94–95
    multitasking and, 96–98
    pets and, 85
    planning ahead and, 114
    positive outlook and, 44
    questionnaire for, 92–94
    relationships and, 62, 65
    and saying "no," 98–101
    setting goals for dealing with, 261–62
    sleep and, 104–6
    sound and, 118
    stretching and, 155
    tai chi and, 155
    at work, 62, 109–12
    see also relaxation
stress hormones, 62, 90–91, 102, 103, 114, 121
stretching, 150, 151–52, 217
    balance and flexibility work, 7, 149, 154–57, 158, 160, 217
    flexibility and strengthening workout, 161–82
    at work, 111
stroke, 188, 210, 216, 218
    anger and, 102
    diet and, 192, 194
    exercise and, 145
    gum disease and, 246
    omega-3 fats and, 192, 231
    smoking and, 135
    stress and, 91, 110
    workplace and, 110
sulfonylurea drugs, 218
sun exposure, 136, 236